AF589380

A Systematic Guide for Microbial Identification

The Authors

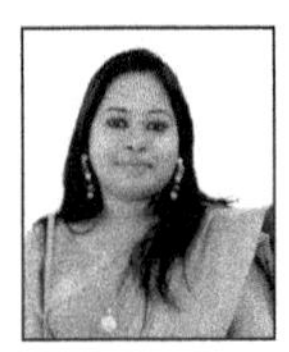

Dr Shubhashree Mahalik is Assistant Professor at P.G. Department of Biosciences and Biotechnology, Fakir Mohan University, Balasore, Odisha. She holds MSc degree in Biotechnology from University of Allahabad and PhD degree in Biotechnology from Jawaharlal Nehru University. She specializes in Microbial Bioprocess and biosystems engineering. Her doctoral research work focused on systems biology approaches for designing Quiescent cell platform for over expression of recombinant proteins. Presently she is engaged in research work pertaining to study of microbial physiology and metabolic engineering for production of value-added enzymes and metabolites.

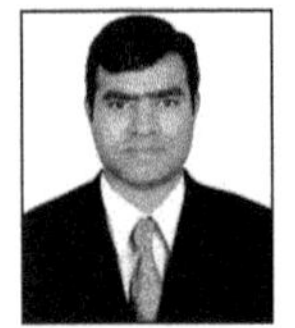

Dr Dhanesh Kumar is currently working as a prestigious Dr. D. S. Kothari Post Doctoral Fellow at Dept. of Plant Sciences, School of Life Sciences, University of Hyderabad, Hyderabad. He has earned his master's and Doctoral degree from Visva-Bharati, Santiniketan, an Institution of national importance. Dr. Kumar served as guest faculty in Fakir Mohan University, Balasore, teaching microbiology and Biotechnology to P.G. and M. Phil students. His present research thrust includes study of diversity of bacteria in coastal belt of Odisha, isolation of novel phylotypes and metagenome analysis. Dr. Kumar is the recipient of international fellowship from Govt. of Czech Republic, National merit scholarship from DBT, Govt. of India, CSIR-NET, ICMR JRF, GATE etc.

A Systematic Guide for Microbial Identification

Dr Shubhashree Mahalik
Dr Dhanesh Kumar

2019
Daya Publishing House®
A Division of
Astral International Pvt. Ltd.
New Delhi – 110 002

ISBN: 9789390384587 (HB)

Published by : **Daya Publishing House®**
A Division of
Astral International Pvt. Ltd.
– ISO 9001:2015 Certified Company –
4736/23, Ansari Road, Darya Ganj
New Delhi-110 002
Ph. 011-43549197, 23278134
E-mail: info@astralint.com
Website: www.astralint.com

Digitally Printed at : **Replika Press Pvt. Ltd.**

Preface

Microbiology has always been a fascinating subject for students and researchers. The domain of Microbiology is quite vast and comprises the study of microbial diversity, morphology, physiology, pathology, genetics, evolution as well as food and industrial microbiology. Therefore it is essential to isolate and identify the microorganisms before studying it in details. The book, A Systematic Guide for Microbial Identification introduces the basic yet essential techniques used for isolation and identification of microorganisms. This book is designed for science and medical graduate, post graduates and research scholars who are new to the field of microbiology.

The book is designed in a simple, concise manner having easy protocols and diagrams for better understanding. Several microscopic, biochemical, staining as well as genetic and advanced tools and techniques have been compiled to make this book a one stop solution for microbial identification.

The basic idea was to make a comprehensive book that can be widely used for better understanding of microbial world. The language and content has been kept simple in order to make it interesting, convenient and accessible. We hope the students will appreciate the book and will justify its name of being the best guide for Systematic identification of microbes.

The authors acknowledge their respective host institutions for providing support in the preparation of this book.

Authors

Abbreviations

2D	Two dimension
3D	Three dimension
CCD	Charge-Coupled device
CLSM	Confocal laser scanning microscope
CO_2	Carbon dioxide
CRF	Coagulase reacting factor
CV-I	Crystal Violet Iodine (CV-I) complexes
DMSO	Dimethyl sulfoxide
DNA	Deoxyribonucleic acid
FACS	Fluorescence-activated cell sorting
FAME	Fatty Acid Methyl Ester
FISH	Fluorescent *in situ* hybridization
FITC	Fluorescein-5-isothiocyanate
FSC	Forward scatter
GC	*Guanine+Cytosine* content
GRD	Genomic based 16S Ribosomal RNA Database
HCl	Hydrochloric acid
HPLC	High-performance liquid chromatography
HRM	High Resolution Melting
LCSM	Laser confocal scanning microscope
LD_{50}	Lethal dose
LED	Light-emitting diode
LPCB	Lactophenol cotton blue
MIC	Minimum inhibitory concentration
NaCl	Sodium chloride
NaOH	Sodium hydroxide

NGS	Next Generation Sequencing
nm	Nanometre
NO_2	Nitrogen dioxide
OTU	Operational Taxonomic Units
PBS	Phosphate-buffered saline
PCR	Polymerase Chain Reaction
pH	Power of hydrogen/ Potential of hydrogen
PMT	Photomultiplier tubes
RAPD	Random Amplified Polymorphic DNA
RDP	Ribosomal Database Project
RFLP	Restriction Fragment Length Polymorphism
RNA	Ribonucleic acid
rRNA	Ribosomal RNA
SEM	Scanning Electron Microscope
SNPs	Single Nucleotide Polymorphisms
SOP	Standard Operating Procedure
SSC	Side-scattered
TEM	Transmission Electron Microscopy
T_m	Melting temperature
UV	Ultra violet

Contents

Chapter

1

Introduction

The diverse world of microbes is engrossing and captivating. Microbes include organisms that are of micron size, not visible to naked eye and can only be seen under microscope. They are the first life form on this earth and appeared around 3 billion years ago. The microbes are unicellular organism having either prokaryotic or eukaryotic type of cell organization. Till 17th century scientific world was unaware of microbial world. Antonie Philips van Leeuwenhoek, a Dutch tradesman and scientist, observed several materials and communicated the findings to Royal Society in London. His discovery of "animalcules" brought into light a different world.

Every strata of our ecosystem is populated with thousands and thousands of microbial species. Microbes can be our friends as well as foes. They are directly as well as indirectly linked to our everyday life. Some may be pathogenic and infectious whereas others are beneficial as they are fixer of CO_2, NO_2 participate in bioremediation of the toxic wastes, enhance soil fertility, decompose and degrade the carcasses of animals. They are also a potential source drugs, food and fuel supplements. Out of this diverse world very few bacteria (0.1 to 1 %) have been identified due to the inability to culture them in laboratory condition and a large population still lies unexplored. Therefore there has been a surge in development of tools and techniques to isolate and identify this unexplored territory.

Microbial taxonomy is one of the oldest branches of science with more than 250-year-old history. It is a method of grouping microbes on the basis of certain selected common characters. Taxonomy includes three aspects i.e. classification (arrange organisms into groups called taxa), nomenclature (assignment of names to taxonomic groups as per standard practice) and identification (determination of typical characters of the isolate and assignment of taxon).

While previous classification was primarily based on phenotypic characters like cell shape, cell size, presence of cilia and flagella, cellular inclusions, colour, mechanism of motility, endospore shape and location, spore morphology and location, colony morphology, ultra structural characteristics, staining behavior etc. It later included physiological, metabolic and ecological characteristics like general nutritional type, requirement of carbon and nitrogen sources, energy sources, mechanisms of energy conversion, cell wall constituents, fermentation products, luminescence, motility, osmotic tolerance, growth temperature optimum and range, pH optimum and growth range, photosynthetic pigments, salt requirements and tolerance, secondary metabolites formed, sensitivity to metabolic inhibitors and antibiotics etc. This system of classification is termed as Phenetic classification. The second aspect is phylogenetic classification, where the microbes are classified on the basis of their evolutionary relationships. Phylogenetic classification largely based on the genetic and molecular characteristics of the microbes. In this technique molecular aspect like GC content, nucleotide sequencing (16s rRNA), nucleic acid hybridization, amino acid composition, protein profiling, enzymatic activity, metabolite production are considered for exploring the phylogenetic linkage between various groups of microbes. But a complete understanding of a microbe requires both phenetic and phylogenetic characterization.

Modern approaches like next generation sequencing, whole genome sequencing, DNA microarray, metagenomics, proteomics, metabolomics etc are rapidly used. But they are costly and require specific instrumentation and expertise. Therefore it is advisable to use basic tools and techniques for phenetic and phylogenetic characterization that could be followed by modern approaches.

The chapters in this book discuss the various classical as well as modern methods and techniques for identification of microbial isolate. The book begins with a chapter of general instructions that needs to be followed in a Microbiology laboratory and is very essential to successfully perform microbial experiments. Chapter 3 discusses principle, types and application of microscopy which is a very important instrument in the study of microbiology. Media is critical for growth and culture of microbes and therefore a brief idea regarding the types of culture media used in microbiology are discussed in Chapter 4. In Chapter 5 various culture techniques are discussed which helps us to grow microbes in our desired culture media. Once we have obtained microbial culture, it is very essential to study its growth kinetics, therefore in Chapter 6 various methods have been discussed to study the growth profile of microbes. Apart from growth and culturing of microbes it is very crucial to know the method of preservation of microbes that has been discussed in Chapter 7. Once the microbes are in culturable condition, it is necessary to study its characteristics. The primary identification begins with morphological characterization of microbial colonies. So Chapter 8 discusses typical colony characters. Following this several staining methods are discussed in Chapter 9 to observe microbial morphology under microscope. Chapter 10 discusses the Biochemical tests that are performed to screen and identify microbes on the basis of their response to biochemical tests. Chapter 11 discusses the advanced molecular technique which uses biomolecules like DNA, RNA, proteins and fatty acids to profile the microbes on the basis of the changes in the bimolecular characteristics. Finally Chapter 12 discusses Metagenomics which is one of the advanced techniques for identification and phylogenetic classification of microbial communities containing both culturable and unculturable microbes.

Chapter

2

General Laboratory Instruction

1. In any experiment, data compilation is very important. Therefore a laboratory data notebook should be kept for compiling all observations during the experimental procedure. The notebook should be well maintained and up to date by the researcher. An index should be prepared where all experiments performed should be entered date wise.
2. Before the start of the experiment all information related to the experiment should be noted down like the, title of the experiment, principle of the experiment, chemicals and instruments required as well as the detailed protocol, experimental conditions, total time required to complete the experiment and the recipe of all the chemicals and buffers prepared.
3. If any biological samples are involved in the experiment all the information related to it like the source, genotype, accession number of the dataset, storage conditions, contagious or safe, handling instructions should be enlisted in the notebook.
4. A result section should be included where all the observations and raw data should be noted down. All drawings, diagrams, graphs and tables related to the data should be included in this section.
5. An indent of all the materials required in lab should be prepared which could include sections like biological as well as non-biological materials, hazardous and non-hazardous chemicals, molecular biology grade reagents, microbiology related reagents, tissue culture grade reagents etc. The articles listed in the indent should comprise of information like source, supplier, date of purchase, date of expiry, number of units present, storage conditions, concentration and any other special instructions.
6. All chemicals used in the laboratory must be handle carefully. Before using any chemical the Material Safety Data Sheets should be examined carefully and all the instructions should be followed precisely.
7. While handling hazardous chemicals proper protection should be taken like laboratory coat, gloves, face mask and, eye gear should be worn. Mouth pipetting should also be avoided.

8. In case of any spillage or accidental exposure, the concerned authority should be immediately informed and adequate steps should be taken to clean the spillage or rescue the persons involved in the accident.
9. Instruments are an integral part of every laboratory. They should be well maintained and handled carefully. Indents should also be prepared for all instruments. They should be maintained in working condition and annual maintenance information should be well recorded.
10. An SOP should be prepared for all the instruments. For high end specialized instruments concerned technicians should be hired to operate and maintain the instrument. Before using any instrument, the technician in charge should be consulted, if needed it should be calibrated and operated according to SOP.
11. A log book entry should be made before using the instruments. Any error during operation should be immediately reported or mentioned in the remarks section of the log book.
12. Glass and plastic wares used for experimental works must be properly cleaned. Glassware should be cleaned with mild detergent, rinsed with distilled water followed by autoclaving, drying or baking in a hot oven at high temperature. Glass wares used for molecular biology works should be pretreated to make them free from proteinase and pyrogens. Similarly plastic ware, pipettes, culture tubes microtips, and microcentrifuge tubes should be autoclaved or presterilized plastic wares should be purchased.
13. Preparation of stock solutions and reagents is a critical step of every experiment. Therefore extra care should be taken in calculations which includes molarity/normality, percent calculation and other calculations. It is preferred to maintain a chart where calculations for all stock solutions are done already. This would minimize errors that could occur during miscalculations. Similarly all important formulae could also be enlisted for reference during experiments.
14. Another parameter which is essential during stock preparation is the accurate weighing of chemicals. For this precise weighing balance should be used. The weighing balance should be calibrated time to time.
15. After preparation of stock solutions it should be accordingly sterilized either by autoclaving or membrane filtration. If the solution requires a specific pH, then it should be checked by accurate pH meter and maintained accordingly by either addition of 2N NaOH or 2N HCl.
16. Storage of stock solutions is again critical. Storage temperature and duration should be checked for each solution. Date of preparation and date of expiry for each solution should be mentioned on the storage bottle. Some chemicals are light sensitive and therefore they could be prepared and stored in dark bottles and placed in such a way that they do not get exposed to light.

17. Before using any chemical it should be checked for expiry date, contamination or degradation. In this case it should be immediately disposed and fresh solution should be prepared.
18. Disposal of buffer, chemicals and culture media should be specially taken care of. Specified discard bins should be provide in the laboratory for disposal of hazardous and nonhazardous discards as well as for biological and non-biological items. Biological items should be autoclaved before disposal. No laboratory chemical should be directly discarded in the sink. Radioactive waste and animal carcasses should be disposed as per ethical committee guidelines.
19. Ultraviolet light is used in laminar air flows and incubators for disinfection as well as in UV-transilluminators for visualization of DNA. Extensive exposure to UV light can cause eye irritation and damage to retina.
20. Formaldehyde fumigation is one of the oldest methods of laboratory disinfection. It is a cost effective methods and microbiologically recognized method, but formaldehyde is a toxic chemical which causes eye & nose irritation and it is also known to be a potential carcinogen. Therefore care must be taken before handling formaldehyde. The concerned persons should be provided with personal protective equipments. A warning must be issued during the fumigation procedure.
21. Electrical connections and all circuits should be well maintained. They should be regularly checked. Since all equipments run on electricity, any fluctuations in voltage or current can damage the equipment as well as cause electrocution, which could be lethal.
22. Proper fire safety measures should be taken in the laboratory. Fire extinguisher, fire alarm box and emergency exit plans should be well places in the laboratories. They should be checked at regular intervals and fire safety trainings should be given to researchers. Flammable and combustible chemicals should be carefully stored at an isolated place.
23. First aid box should be readily available in laboratories.
24. General Housekeeping plan should be streamlined. The laboratory area and working bench should be free of clutter. Discard bins should be cleaned every day. No electrical wires should lie on the floor and it should be properly grounded. All refrigerators, storage boxes and shelves should be properly labelled and indents should be maintained for each segment. There should be a daily laboratory cleaning plan and monthly laboratory disinfection plan to avoid contaminations and accidents.
25. Finally there should be laboratory meetings at frequent intervals where laboratory management issues should be discussed and problems should be addressed.

Chapter 3

Microscope and its Handling

Microscope is the mother of microbiology. A microscope is a tool to visualize the small objects which are difficult to see with naked eyes. The microscope has introduced us to a new dimension of lives that are present around us but are not known, due to the inability of human eye to see this. The credit for inventing first microscope is given to Antonie Van Leeuwenhoek, a Dutch draper and scientist. Leeuwenhoek who made a single lens microscope was able to magnify the objects 20-40 folds. Later he improved his microscopes with several combinations and was able to magnify the objects by more than 250x. It has been also claimed that double lens microscope (compound microscope) was invented by Zacharias Jansen and his father during 1590s, much before the Leeuwenhoek.

Microscope is a great tool for visualizing, identifying and characterizing a microbe. Microbial identification using microscope is the most traditional ways of studying microbes. Microbes are identified based on their morphological character as well as physiological behavior.

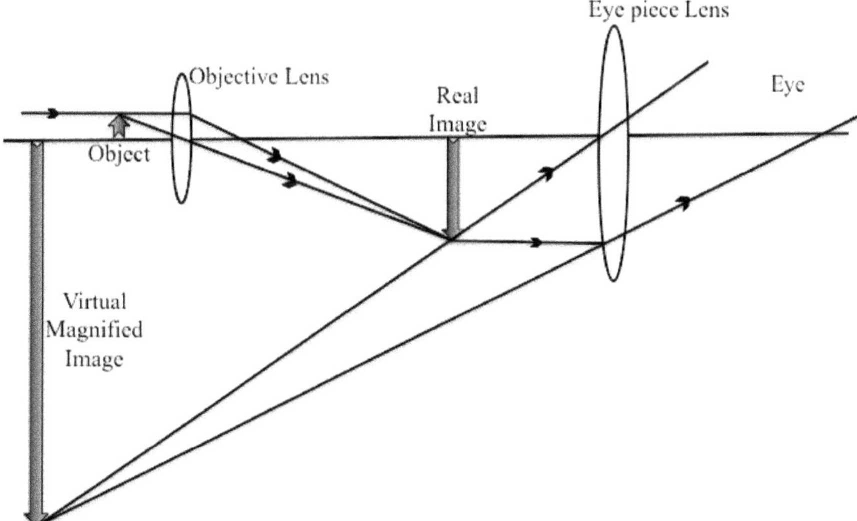

Fig. 3.1: Ray diagram of image formation by a simple (compound) microscope.

Principle

Microscope uses the magnifying power of lenses. In microscope, one or more lenses are arranged in specific manner to enlarge the image of an object which has to be observed. Generally two lenses are required for image formation. One lens is near to object and is known as objective whereas the lens nearer to eye is known as eyepiece. The light coming from the object passes through the objective and makes a magnified real and inverted image of the object. This inverted image is again magnified by eyepiece which is virtual and upright. This virtual image is seen by eyes through eyepiece.

Microscope used in microbial identification

1. Compound Microscope

Compound microscope is the general yet effective microscope used in common practical laboratories. A compound microscope has an objective, an eyepiece, a revolving nosepiece, stage, curved arm, two knobs for coarse adjustment and fine adjustment, a light source, condenser and the base. Revolving nosepiece which contains 3-4 objective lenses with different magnification power usually 4x, 10x, 40x and 100x. Modern compound microscope has inbuilt facility of light whose intensity can be controlled whereas in older version mirrors are used for collecting light. Condenser concentrates the light which fall on the object and through object enters into objective. To see an object or microbe, it should be mounted on the slide and the slide should be placed on stage. First the coarse adjustment is used to focus the object then fine adjustment is used to fine tune the image. To select the area on the slide where our object is present, first we use 4x magnification lens as it covers a large slide area. The area is selected and objective of higher magnification is used gradually to see the enlarged image of the object. For higher magnification usually more than 40x, immersion oil is used between slide and objective. The oil has almost the same refractive index as glass (1.5) which prevents the refraction of light which occurs in presence of air (refractive index 1) between slide and objective. A compound microscope can magnify an object image as much as 1000x.

2. Fluorescence Microscope

Certain chemicals when illuminated with light of certain wavelength, start emitting light of higher wavelength (lower energy than the incident light). These chemicals are known as fluorophore and this phenomenon is known as fluorescence. Fluorescent microscope uses this phenomenon. The fluorescent microscope can be defined as the microscope which uses the fluorescence or phosphorescence to generate the image of the specimen that has to be visualized. To generate the image of the specimen, first it has to be stained with fluorophore. Common fluorophores used for staining the specimen are acridine orange, acridine yellow, thioflavin, 4′, 6-diamidino-2-phenylindole (DAPI) etc. Some marine organisms also produce certain proteins which shows fluorescence e.g. Green fluorescence protein (GFP) produced by *Aequorea victoria*, a jelly fish.

The fluorescence microscope contains a strong light source, excitation filter, dichroic mirror or dichroic beam splitter and emission filter or barrier filter as their main component. Light source may be xenon arc lamp, mercury lamp, high power LED or laser in some advance version of microscope. Light source generally produce white light which is the mixture of light of different colors. Excitation filter screen this light and allow only the blue light to pass through it. This blue light passes through objective and illuminates the specimen. The specimen, stained with fluorescent dye absorbs this blue light and emits the light of higher wavelength (mostly green colored light). This light goes upward and passes through objective and dichroic mirror. This mirror allows only green light to pass through it and reflect the light of other wavelength, if any. Now the light passes through the barrier filter or emission filter which again allow only green light to pass through it and block any light of other wavelength which might have not reflected by dichroic mirror. Now we perceive the image of the specimen which is stained by fluorescence dye in green colour. The unstained portion of the specimen remains invisible. The light coming from light source to excite the specimen and the fluorescent light emitted by specimen use the same path i.e. through objective. Since the light is coming from above to excite the specimen, this fluorescence microscope is also known as epifluorescence microscope. This is the common fluorescence microscope used biological laboratories.

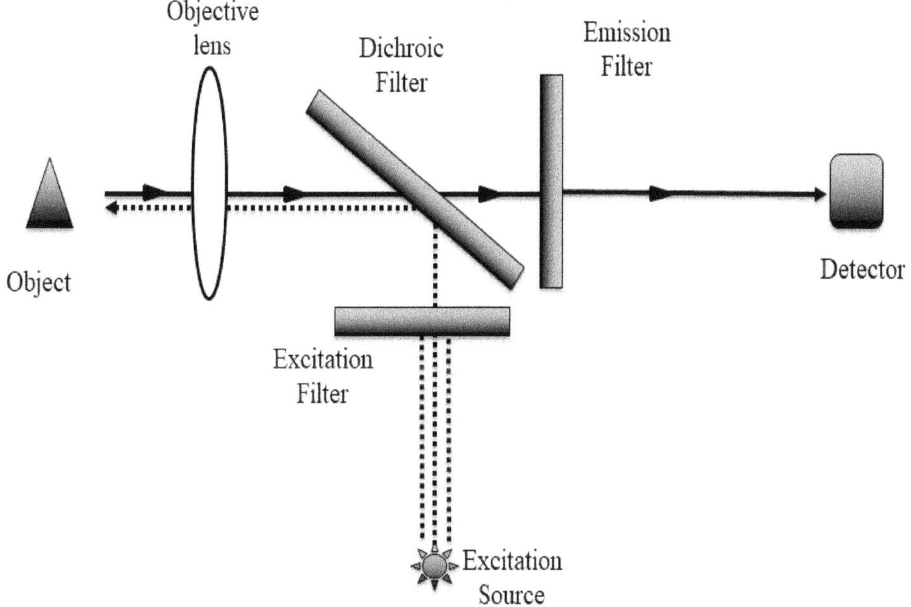

Fig. 3.2: Ray diagram of fluorescent microscope.

3. Confocal Laser Scanning Microscope (CLSM)

The basic principle of image formation in Confocal laser scanning microscope (CLSM) or laser confocal scanning microscope (LCSM) is same as fluorescence microscope but it uses a spatial pinhole to block the out of the focus rays and allow passage of only focused rays coming from specimen to form the image. This allow better signal to noise ratio and a sharp and contrast image formation of an object or specimen as out of the focus rays are responsible for blurred image formation. In contrast to the fluorescent microscope where the specimen as a whole is illuminated at a time and photodetector or camera form the focused and unfocused image at a time, the CLSM forms the image of focused part of the specimen which is a very tiny part of the specimen (point illumination). Thus it forms several images of the different parts of the specimen at different depth and merge images to form a complete 2D or 3D focused, contrast image. In CLSM, the point illumination and the pinhole are on the same plane in front of detector, from which the name confocal has been derived.

The specimen is scanned by light beam on horizontal plane by multiple oscillating mirrors in x-and y- axis. The scanning speed may vary. Slower scanning speed results in better image formation. As much of the fluorescent light coming from the sample is blocked by the pinhole, the increased resolution is achieved at the cost of decreased light intensity coming to detector. For this reason, sometimes longer exposure time is required. The detector is a photomultiplier tube (PMT) or avalanche photodiode which converts light intensity into electrical signal which is recorded by the computer. Special software is used to decode these signals and form the image.

4. Phase Contrast Microscope

Phase Contrast Microscope is largely used to see the transparent and colorless specimen such as living bacteria in the culture, sub cellular particles, lithographic patterns etc. It enhances the contrast of the object by influencing the light path. The speed of the light becomes slow when it travels through the transparent microbes as compared to the undisturbed light. This creates a difference in the phase of the light. This phase difference is not detected by naked eyes. This difference in phase is increased by half a wavelength by transparent phase plate present in the microscope thus causing a change in brightness. One of the important advantages of phase contrast microscope is that we can see the microbes in natural living condition without killing, fixing or staining them. This allows us to observe dynamic biological process such as bacterial cell proliferation, cell division, motion mechanism etc.

5. Electron Microscope

Electron microscope is the type of microscope which uses the beam of electron instead of beam of light. Resolution of an image is directly related to wavelength of irradiation used in formation of image. As the wavelength of moving electron is much shorter than light, the resolution produced by electron microscope is much higher (in nm range) than the microscope based on light for image formation. Electron microscope can magnify an object 2 million times while the finest light microscope can magnify an object up to 2000 times. Electron microscope use electromagnetic and or electrostatic lens system which is analogous to glass lenses used in light microscope and the image formed is detected by an electron detector and not by the eyes as in case of light microscope.

The electromagnetic lens is a type of solenoid through which current can be passed and thus electromagnetic field can be generated. The fast moving electrons pass through the solenoid and colloids with the sample. These moving electrons are very sensitive to magnetic field and are controlled by changing the current flow through solenoid.

Types of electron microscope

1. **Transmission Electron Microscope (TEM)**: In this electron microscope fast moving electron is generated by cathode. This beam of electrons travels through the electromagnetic lens and strike on the specimen. The transmitted electron through the very thin specimen carries the information about the shape, size and topology of the specimen. The spatial variation in the transmitted electron are captured by the objective lens system and can be viewed by directly exposing the photographic plate on transmitted electron or by fluorescence screen or charged couple device (CCD) camera. This recorded image can be reproduced on computer screen. Transmission electron microscope produce 2-D, black and white image.

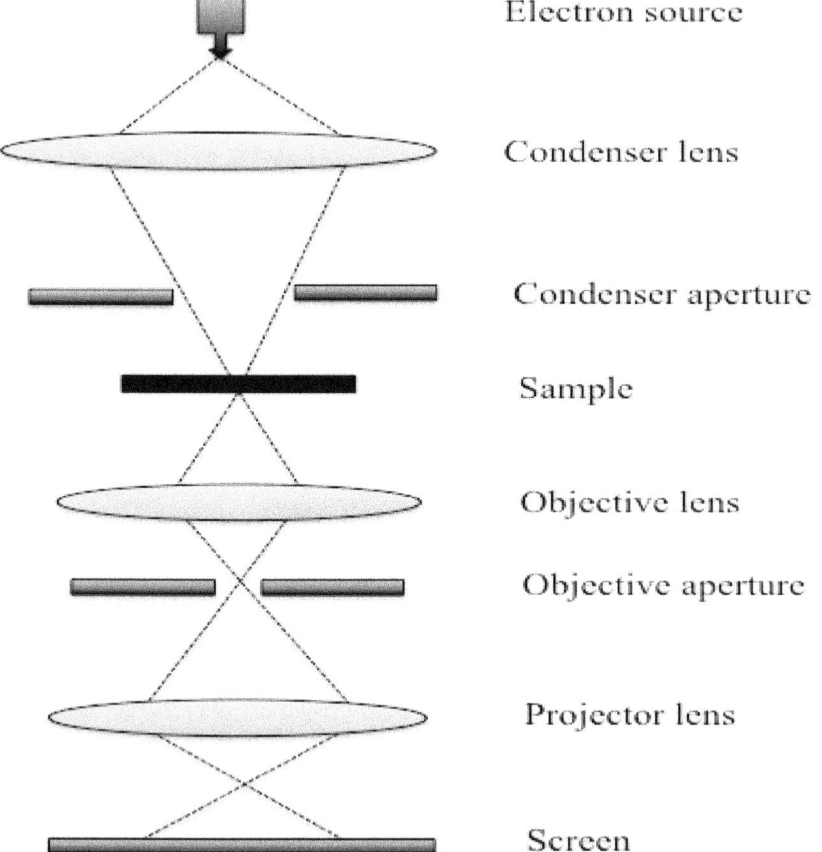

Fig. 3.3: Ray diagram of transmission electron microscope

2. **Scanning Electron Microscope (SEM):** Unlike the TEM in which the image is formed by the transmitted electrons, scanning electron microscope generate image by detecting the low energy secondary electron which are produced when fast moving electron hits the specimen. SEM scan the sample in rectangular manner (raster pattern) and detector build the images by detecting signals with beam position.

   The resolving power of SEM is lower than TEM, however SEM forms the image of sample surface and not the interior of the surface which remove the necessity of forming ultrathin sectioning of sample as it required in TEM.

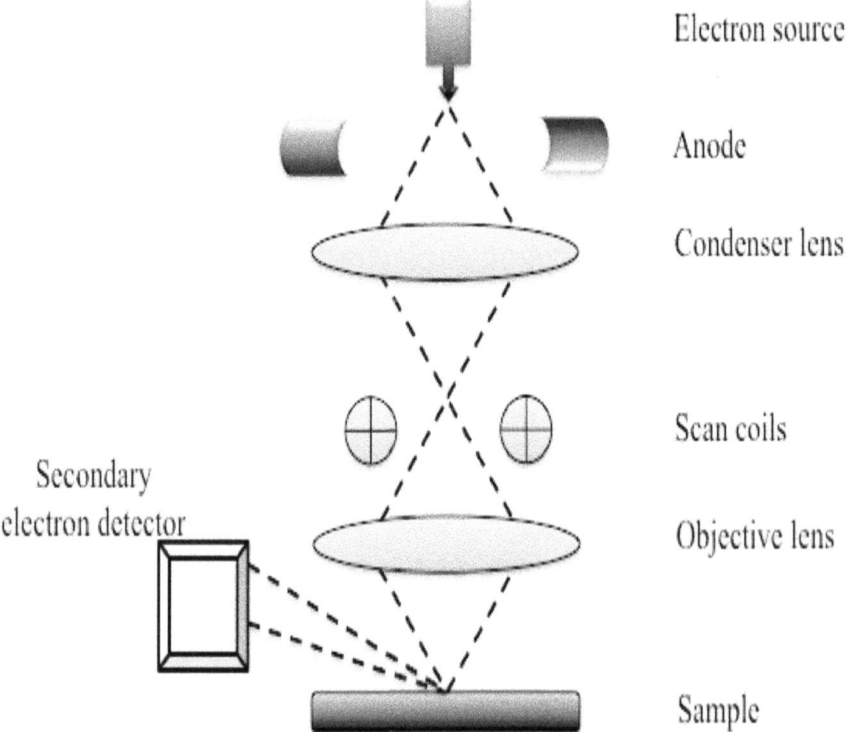

Fig. 3.4: Ray diagram of scanning electron microscope

Handling and Maintenance of Microscope

Microscope is a very sensitive instrument and can go out of order if mishandled or proper care is not taken. Good maintenance of microscope increases its self life and the image quality. The following care must be taken when working with microscope.

1. Microscope must be placed on horizontal and firm bench or table which should be free from any movement or vibration. The working position on microscope should be comfortable.
2. Microscope should be cleaned before and after used. The lenses of the

microscope can easily get scratched. For the same care must be taken during cleaning the lens and it should be cleaned with moist lens paper with lens cleaning solution. Cleaning must be done in circular manner. Use to towel, cotton, tissue paper, water, alcohol etc. to clean the lenses should be avoided.

3. When using the immersion oil, it must be cleaned from the lens immediately after used. Lenses must be dry to avoid any fungal growth over it.
4. Microscope must be covered when not in used to avoid dust accumulation.
5. When working with fluorescent microscope, the lamp must be switched on 5-10 minutes before the use. Once the lamp is switched on, it should not be switched off until 15 minutes. After use, the microscope must be covered when the lamp has been cooled to room temperature.
6. Moving part of the bulb should be lubricated once in a year. The dirt and grease can be removed and a very thin layer of lithium based grease can be applied on the moving parts.
7. Intensity of light used in microscope must be optimum otherwise it can harm observers eye sight.
8. The power connection to microscope and its voltage must be constant and stable.
9. While changing the bulb, use the bulb of appropriate intensity. Bulb inside the microscope must be cooled down before changing. Do not touch the bulb with bare hand.
10. Fluorescent based microscopes should be placed in air conditioned room to easily dissipate the heat generated by the high power light source.

Chapter 4

Culture Media

A culture media otherwise known as growth media is a nutrient source that supports the growth of microorganisms. Culture media is a mixture of macronutrients, micronutrients as well as growth factors. Different microbes have different nutritional requirements and therefore the culture media required for their laboratory propagation also differs.

Types of culture media:

1. On the basis of consistency:

i) **Solid Media:** Contains agar as solidifying agent in the rang of 1-2% agar. Used for isolation of pure culture and study of colony morphology and physiology e.g. Nutrient Agar, Blood Agar.

ii) **Liquid Media:** Does not contain agar. Used for enrichment and mass culture of microbes. Used as suspension culture e.g. Nutrient Broth.

iii) **Semi-solid Media:** Contains 0.5% agar. Used for transportation of microbes or for motility test e.g. Motility medium.

2. On the basis of constituents/ingredients:

i) **Simple/Basal Media:** This is a general purpose media used for growth of microorganisms. It mostly supports non-fastidious bacteria. The composition is very simple comprising of carbon, nitrogen source and buffering agents e.g. Nutrient broth, Nutrient agar.

ii) **Complex Media:** This comprises of basal media to which complex ingredients of biological origin have been added. The complex ingredients are obtained from various species like Yeast extract, Meat extract, Soy extract, brain-heart infusion etc. The exact proportion of these components is not known. Complex media usually provide the full range of growth factors that may be required for cultivation of bacterial pathogens and other fastidious bacteria e.g. Terrific broth, Tryptic Soy agar, Blood agar.

iii) **Synthetic Media:** These types of media are prepared form pure synthetic chemicals. Their exact composition and percentage is known e.g. Peptone water.

iv) Special Media: These groups of media are used for morphological and physiological characterization of microbes. Some of the special media are discussed below:

a) ***Enriched Media:*** In this media, extra nutrients like blood, serum, egg yolk are added to basal medium to make them enriched. Fastidious organisms having special nutritional requirements are grown in this type of media e.g. Blood agar, chocolate agar.

b) ***Selective media:*** This is a differential growth suppression media that selectively suppress the growth of some microorganisms while allowing the growth of others e.g. Thayer Martin agar *(N. gonorrhoeae),* Lowenstein Jensen medium *(M. tuberculosis,)* Potassium tellurite medium *(C. diphtheriae).*

c) ***Enrichment Media:*** It is similar to selective media but used to specifically enhance the concentration or enrich one group of microbes to a detectable level without activating the growth of rest of the bacterial population. It is generally used as broth culture having essential nutrient targeted for the growth of desired microbe e.g. Selenite F broth (*Salmonella, Shigella*), Tetrathionate broth (inhibit coliforms) and alkaline peptone water (*Vibro and cholerae*).

d) ***Indicator Media/Differential Media:*** these media contain certain components like dyes, metabolic substrates that change color on growth of the desired organism. These media allow growth of more than one type of microbial colony and they can be differentiated on the basis of their morphological features due to reaction with incorporated indicators e.g. Wilson-Blair media (*S. typhi* forms black colonies), MacConkey agar (pink colonies by Lactose fermenters).

e) ***Transport Media:*** Used for transportation of microbial samples and clinical isolates. These are generally semi-solid media. They prevent drying, desiccation, contamination and inhibition of growth of microbial samples e.g. Stuart's media.

f) ***Natural Media:*** The media are taken from the site of sampling. It is usually microhabitat of the organism. The soil or water collected from the site of sampling is extracted and filter sterilized and diluted with basal media to grow the organism. The exact composition of this type of media is not known. It is used to grow the bacteria whose exact nutritional requirements are not known. e.g. Coconut water, Ailk, Artificial Sea water.

3. On the basis of Oxygen requirements

*i) **Aerobic media:*** These can be any general purpose liquid media where oxygen is supplied by providing aeration or continuous agitation.

*ii) **Anaerobic media:*** Used for growth of anaerobes. They must have low or no oxygen content. Oxygen is removed by either boiling or by addition of oxidising agents (1% glucose, 0.1% thioglycollate, 0.1% ascorbic acid, 0.05% cysteine or red hot iron filings). Also oxidation-reduction potential indicator is added to the medium e.g. Robertson Cooked meat (*Clostridium* sp.), Thioglycollate broth.

Chapter

5

Culture Techniques

Environmental samples are composed of mixed microbial population such as viruses, bacteria, cyanobacteria, yeast and lower bryophytes. In order to identify and characterize the microbes present in the sample, they have to be isolated into pure culture form. There are several methods which can be applied to obtain pure cultures. In this section these techniques will be discussed. To obtain a pure culture, aseptic conditions must have to be maintained which are outlined in the following section.

Aseptic Conditions

Aseptic technique can be defined as a process of culturing and transferring microorganisms without allowing cross contamination from other unwanted sources. This can be achieved by following these instructions-

1. The work area must be cleaned with 70% ethanol to reduce the number of potential contaminants.
2. The laminar air flow should be exposed to UV radiations for at least 10 minutes before starting any microbiological work.
3. All glass wares and plastic wares to be used should be sterilized by appropriate methods.
4. The inoculating loop should be sterilized by flaming in the blue Bunsen burner before and after using it for transferring of microbial culture.
5. Sterile graduated or dropping (Pasteur) pipettes should be used to transfer cultures, sterile media and sterile solutions. Alternatively autoclavable pipettes can be used.
6. The openings of the bottle and culture tubes should be sterilized by flaming the mouth before inserting your sterile loop into the culture. This decontaminates any unwanted cells that are deposited during the previous experiment.
7. All cultures, chemicals, empty bottles, culture tubes and Petriplates should be kept closed with their respective caps in order to protect them from cross contamination.

8. All culture works need to be done efficiently and quickly in order to prevent exposure to unwanted microbes.

Pure Culture Methods:

1. Streak Plate Method:

This is one of the most common methods used for obtaining pure culture. In this method few drops of mixed microbial population is taken on one side of agar plate and streaked using sterile inoculation loop. 4-5 parallel streaks are made and then the plate is turned 90°C and again the same process is continued touching the last streaked point. Before each round of streaking the loop is sterilized using flame. With each round of streaking the samples get diluted out and in the last section isolated colonies appear.

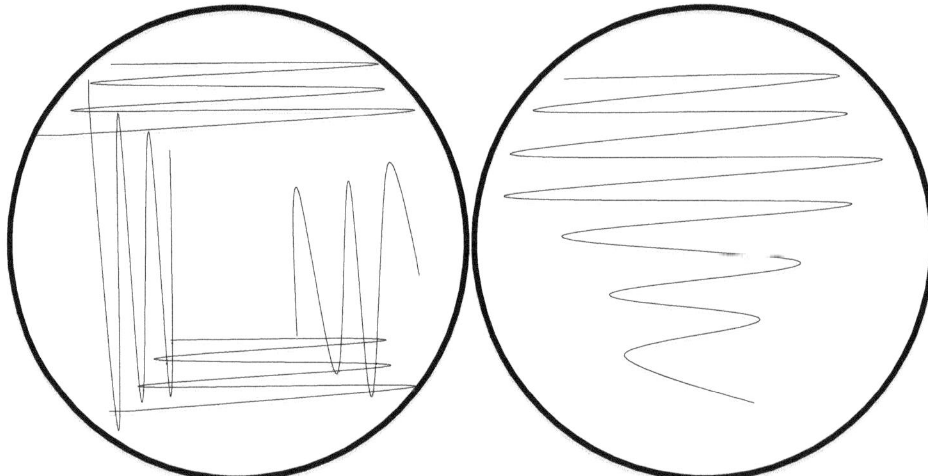

Fig. 5.1: Streak plate method

2. Pour Plate Method:

In this method the mixed microbial population are diluted in appropriate media with molten agar and poured into sterile Petri plates. One part of microbial culture is mixed with 9 parts of molten agar (40-42°C) and mixed uniformly and poured into Petri plates. This method has an advantage that it can be used for isolating and growing both oxygenic and anoxygenic bacteria. Oxygenic will grow over the surface of agar being in contact with air whereas anoxygenic bacteria will grow in embedded condition inside agar. This method has few disadvantages too. Firstly, it is very critical to maintain the temperature of molten agar, because at higher temperature the microbes may get killed and at lower temperature the agar may get solidified prior to dilution of culture. Secondly, sometimes it becomes difficult to isolate the embedded colony using inoculation loop. For isolation of obligate anaerobic bacteria a thick layer (2-5 mm) of paraffin wax can be overlayed on the solid surface of agar media. The wax will prevent the contact of air with growing microbes and provide an excellent anaerobic condition.

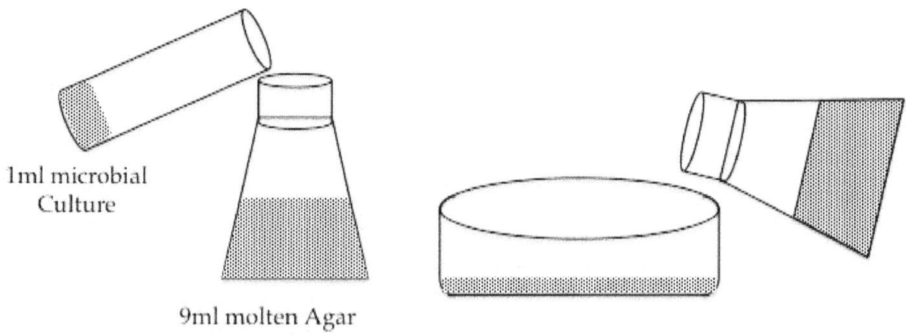

Fig. 5.2: Pour Plate Method

3. Spread Plate method:

In this method the sample is first diluted in sterile media or 1X PBS and , then few drops of diluted samples are placed at the centre of agar plate and then spread onto the agar plate with the help of glass spreader. Glass spreader must be flame sterilized and cooled to ambient temperature to prevent the melting of agar when it come in contact with spreader. Hot spreader may also kill the bacteria present in the sample.

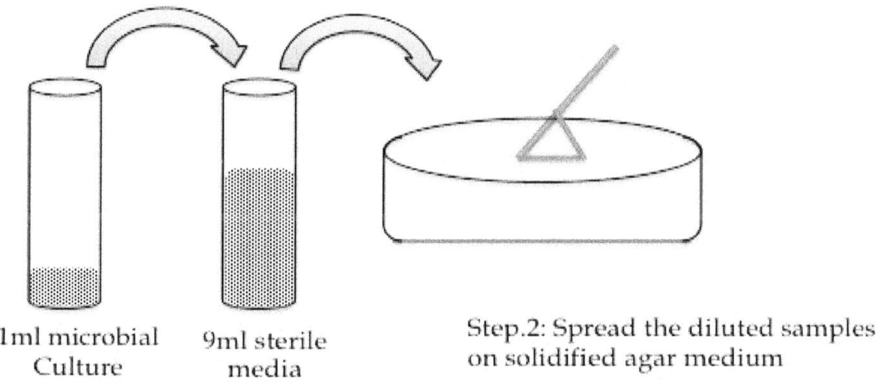

Fig. 5.3: Spread Plate Method

4. Serial dilution Method:

In this method mixed microbial samples are first serially diluted in sterile media or 1X PBS, and the diluted samples are then spread on the agar plates. With each round of dilution the number of population decrease and therefore isolated colonies are obtained.

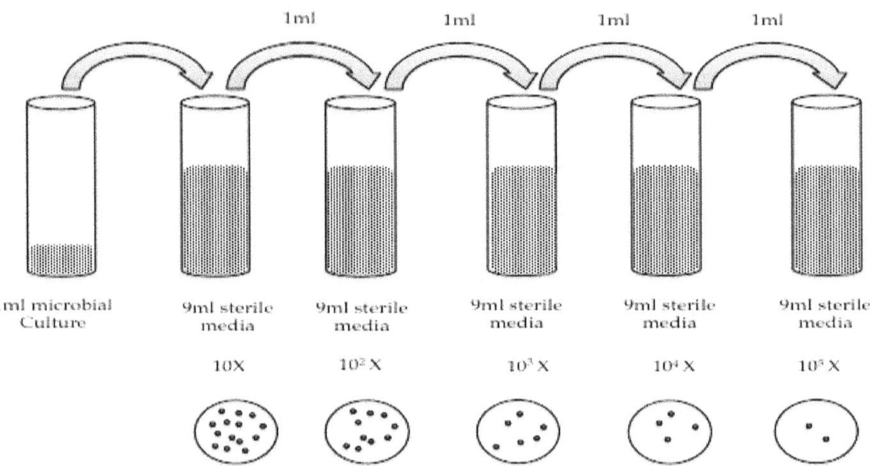

Fig. 5.4: Serial dilutions Method

5. Suspension Culture:

Suspension culture is defined as the system where a single microbial colony multiplies while suspended in liquid medium. This type of culture method is generally used for enrichment or mass culture of microbial cells. Suspension culture can be of various types:

i) **Batch Culture:** These are fixed volume culture conditions where the microbe is grown in suitable nutrient media. Proper physical (temperature, pH, dissolved oxygen) as well as nutrient conditions (media, salinity) are maintained which allows cell propagation. The growth continues till depletion of rate limiting nutrients or change in any physical parameter. To continuously maintain the culture, biomass is measured at regular intervals and as the culture approaches stationary phase they are sub cultured to fresh medium. 1-5% of the densely grown culture can be used to subculture in fresh medium.

ii) **Continuous Culture:** This is a technique where microbial growth take place under a steady state i.e. growth takes place at a fixed specific growth rate under constant environmental conditions. The steady state is maintained by addition of fresh medium and simultaneous removal of old culture at a fixed rate given by the equation

$D=F/V$

D=Dilution rate (h^{-1})

F= Flow rate of media (ml/h)

V=Volume (ml)

The continuous culture could be open type or closed type. In open type the amount of culture removed is replenished by same amount of fresh media. The cells are harvested during removal of culture and the growth is maintained at sub maximal specific growth rate.

In closed continuous culture, fresh medium is added and equal volume of culture is taken out but during removal of culture, the cells are filtered out by mechanical process and only the spent medium is removed. This ensures that the biomass keeps on increasing.

The open type continuous culture is again of two types:

Chemostat: The specific growth rate and overall cell density is fixed at a constant rate by adjusted addition of rate limiting nutrient. The rate of addition of rate limiting nutrient is reflected by the change in the specific growth rate.

Turbidostat: In this method the optical density of the culture is critical. Optical density determines the turbidity of the culture. In turbidostat, the rate of addition of fresh medium is controlled at a fixed optical density (turbidity).

iii) **Fed-batch Culture:** A fed-batch culture is a semi-batch or semi-closed system. In this system the nutrients necessary for cell growth and product formation (carbon, nitrogen, phosphates, nutrients, precursors, or inducers) are fed either intermittently or continuously. The culture broth is harvested usually only at the end of the operation. The feed is designed as per culture conditions and fed as per growth rate of the microbes. The feed can be added either at a constant rate or exponentially matching the specific growth rate. Therefore, the culture volume increases by the end of the operation. Fed-batch culture is designed to increase the concentration of the desired product at the end of the run.

Chapter

6

Estimation of Growth of Microbes

Microbial growth is defined as the increase in population. It has two aspects i.e. increase in number as well as increase in biomass. A typical microbial growth has 4 stages: lag phase, log phase, stationary phase and death phase or decline phase. There are several direct and indirect methods to measure microbial growth. Few of them are discussed in this chapter.

Breed Method

This is a direct method of cell counting. In this method a fixed volume of cell culture is taken, fixed by appropriate method, stained and observed under microscope. Since it is not possible to count each cell in the smear prepared, it is advised to fix few microscopic fields within 1 cm^2 of the smear and count the cells from those fields.

The total number of cells can be counted using the following formulae:

(a)Area of microscopic field = πr^2

r =radius of lens

(b)Area of the smear = 1 cm^2 = 100 mm^2.

No. of microscopic fields = $100/\pi r^2$

(c) No. of cells in 1 cm^2= Average no. of microbes per microscopic field x ($100/\pi r^2$)

Petroff-Hausser Counting Chamber

These are glass slides having special grid lines streaked on it. The grids or the rulings cover 9 square millimeters. Boundary lines of the Neubauer ruling are the center lines of the groups of three. The central square millimeter is ruled into 25 groups of 16 small squares, each group separated by triple lines, the middle one of which is the boundary. The ruled surface is 0.02 mm below the cover glass, so that the volume over a square millimeter is 0.02 cubic mm. Count all cells within this center square millimeter (1mm x 1mm area). The squares that are 1/400 mm^2 in area; a glass cover slip rests 1/50 mm above the slide, so that the volume over a square is 1/20,000 mm^3 (i.e., 1/20,000,000 cm^3). A bacterial culture is diluted and place on this grid area and counted under microscope.

The total number of cells can be counted using the following formulae:

No. of cells counted x 20,000,000 cm^3x dilution

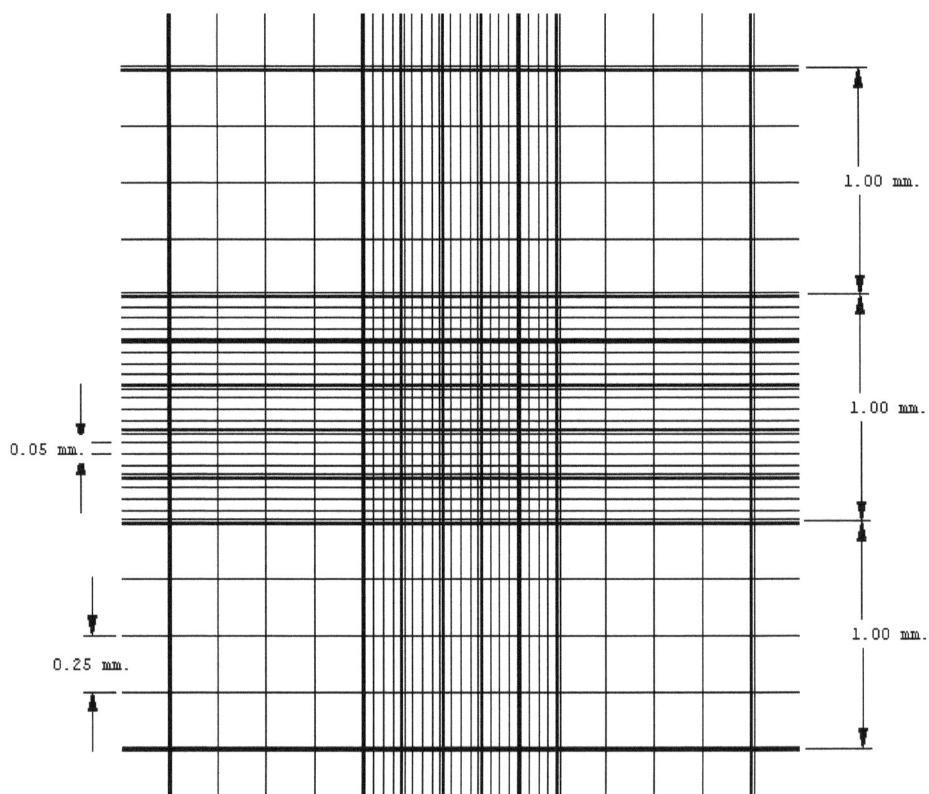

Fig. 6.1: Petroff-Hausser counting chamber

Viable Cell Count

The bacterial culture may not always comprise of live cells. It is basically a mix of dead and live cells. Unless the live cells are stained with appropriate dye they cannot be directly counted under microscope by methods described in previous sections. Therefore alternative methods have been designed to specifically count viable cells. One of the simplest methods is to count the number of colonies developed on nutrient agar plate. The hypothesis behind this method is that only a viable cell with a normal physiology would be able to produce colonies when grown on appropriate media. Therefore the microbial samples are serially diluted in phosphate buffered saline (1: 10, 1: 100, 1: 1000, 1: 10,000, and 1: 1,000,00) and 1 ml of each dilution is spread over agar medium by pour plate method or spread plate method. The plates are allowed to incubate for appropriate time duration at appropriate temperature. Post incubation, the number of colonies appeared on the plates are counted.

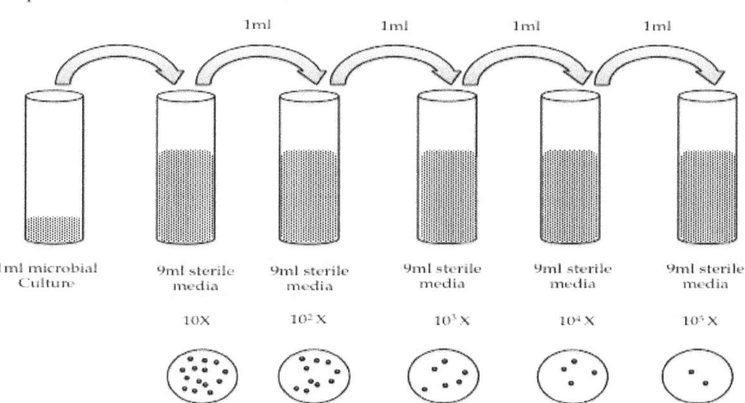

Fig. 6.2: Schematic representation of cell counting by viable count method

The total number of cells can be counted using the following formulae:

No. of colonies counted x dilution x volume of sample plated

Membrane Filter Method

This is one of the oldest and simplest methods for counting number of viable cells. In this technique samples are filtered through membrane filters due to which microbes of different sizes are trapped in the pores of membrane filters. This membrane filter is then transferred onto solidified agar plate. The plates are incubated and number of colonies appeared on the plate is counted. Since microbes of various size can get trapped in the pores of membrane filter, therefore post incubation we can observe diverse colonies on agar plates. We can selectively grow few microbes by incubating the filter paper on selective media, or by changing the incubation time and temperature.

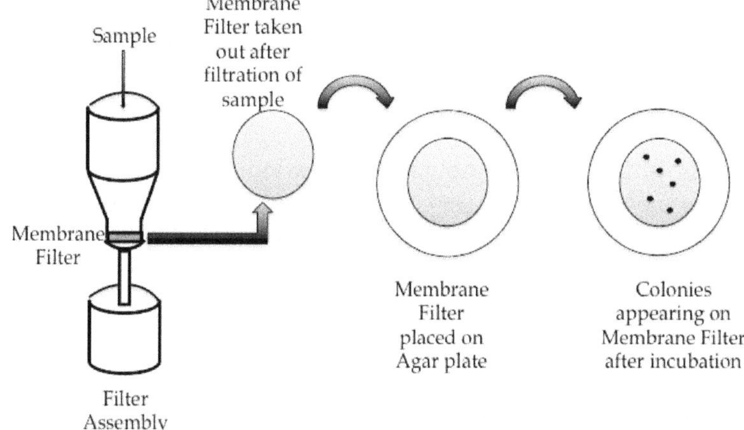

Fig. 6.3: Schematic representation of cell counting by Membrane Filter method

Coulter Counter

The Coulter counter is one of the oldest method to count particles of various sized on the basis of changes in the electrical impedance produced by these nonconductive particles suspended in an electrolyte. The instrument consists of two electrodes and a small aperture passing through the electrode. The size of the aperture is such that only one particle can escape through the aperture. This mechanism is presently used for counting cells suspended in a solution. When a bacterial cell passes through the aperture electrical resistance between the two electrodes increases momentarily or the conductivity drops. This generates an electrical signal, which is automatically counted. Each such electrical signal counts for one bacterial cell.

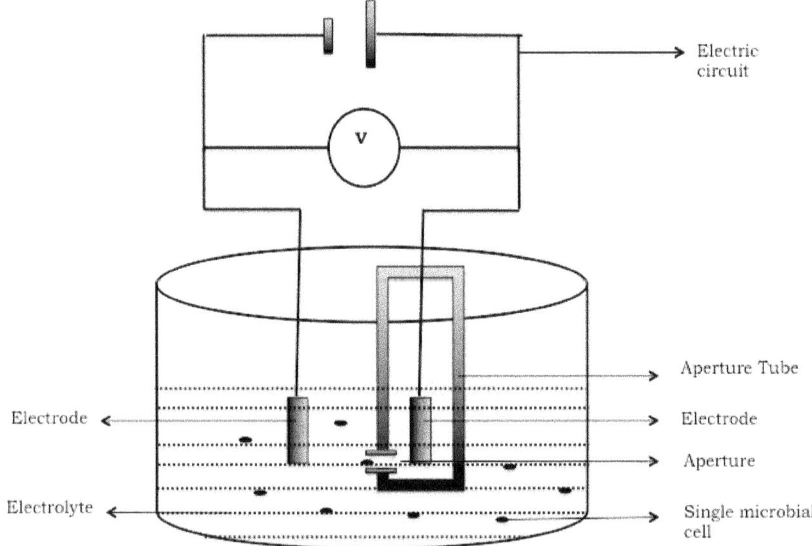

Fig. 6.4: Schematic representation of Coulter Counter

Measurement of cell population by turbidometric method

In a spectrophotometer cell number or density can be determined by measuring the scattering of light by individual cells. Since in a homogeneous population, size of each microbe would be same, therefore increase in scattering is directly proportional to increase in cell number. The microbial suspension culture appears to be dense or turbid after few hours of incubation. This is due to the increase in cell population. So turbidity is used as a parameter for direct measurement of cell density. Higher the turbidity, lower is the transmission of light, greater is the cell density.

Measurement of cell mass by dry weight

In this method, the cells are filtered from the suspension culture and put in a pre-weighted glass bottle. The sample is then placed in a desiccator to remove the moisture. After the cells have dried they are again weighed and the dry mass of the cell population is estimated.

Chapter 7

Preservation of Microbes

One critical aspect of microbiology is the art of preservation of microbes. Different microbes have different growth rate and different life span. Unless preserved appropriately there is every chance of losing the viability of the microbial isolate. Also it is necessary to maintain the purity of the isolate and keep it free from contamination. During day to day experimental work it is advisable to subculture the microbial culture to maintain its viability. But if the number of isolate is very high, handling and sub culturing of such a large collection becomes difficult. Although sub culturing is done in an aseptic environment, but with each sub culturing, the risk of contamination increases. Also as the cells are maintained in an active and dividing stage, the accumulation of mutations with each cell division cycle increases. So with the increase in number of generations, the number of mutations also increases. These factors therefore demands for designing strategies to store microbes in a metabolically inactive but viable condition. Few commonly used strategies that are commonly used in laboratories for storage of microbes are discussed here.

Refrigeration

In this technique the microbes are stored at 4°C. Storing at 4°C ensures that the enzymes become inactive at this temperature which renders the microbe metabolically inactive. General refrigerators are used for this type of storage. To store microbes through refrigeration, they have to be either spread or streaked on Nutrient agar plates, or inoculated on agar slants. These plates or slants are incubated at appropriate temperature and once visible growth is achieved, they are place in refrigerators. Care must be taken for proper sealing of the plates and slants to avoid contamination and drying of media. Plates are sealed with Parafilm whereas slants are prepared in glass culture tubes having screw caps. Also agar stabs can be prepared in micro centrifuge tubes by adding 1ml of melted Nutrient agar into sterile micro centrifuge tubes and allow them to solidify. Once solidified a single colony can be inoculated using a needle. These types of stabs are used for short term storage. By refrigeration bacteria can be stored for 2-3 weeks while fungi can be stored for 3-4 months.

2. Paraffin Method

This is the most simplest method for storage of pure cultures. In this method melted paraffin is poured over agar plates or slants and kept in an upright position. Paraffin prevents drying of media, also its provides anaerobic environment where the metabolic activity of the microbes slows down. By this method the microbes can be stored for several months.

3. Freezing

This is also a method of storage at ultra low temperature. The cultures are kept in a frozen condition at temperature ranging from -20°C to -80°C. There are Laboratory freezers (-20°C to -40°C) and ultra low freezers (-80°C) where these temperature can be maintained. But the major problem with ultra low temperature is the formation of ice crystals within the cell which ruptures the cell membrane and cell wall and may lead to cell lysis. As the water gets converted to ice, the amount of salt concentration increases within the cytoplasm due to dehydration and high salt concentration may lead to damage of various biomolecules. To avoid these problems cryoprotectants like glycerol and DMSO are used. Glycerol or DMSO in the range of 5% to 15% can be added to microbial cultures before preserving them under ultra low condition. In this method microbes can be stored for years.

4. Cryopreservation

This is a very sensitive method where microbes are stored at -196°C. For this method liquid nitrogen is required. Also this method demands special cryovials and cryogenic storage units. This is an expensive method as liquid nitrogen is not readily available everywhere. Glycerol or DMSO in the range of 5% to 15% are used as cryoprotectants.

5. Lyophilization

This method is also known as Freeze drying method. Freeze-drying is a process where water and other solvents are removed from a frozen product via sublimation. In this method, the culture is rapidly frozen at a very low temperature (-70°C) and then dehydrated by vacuum. Under these conditions, the microbial cells are dehydrated and they become metabolically inactive; as a result, the microbes are in a dormant state and therefore can be stored for several years without compromising on their viability. This is also an expensive method as specialized instruments are required for freeze drying. But the microbial cells can be stored for more than 10 years.

Quality Control After Preservation

When the microbial isolates are taken out from storage for experimental work few, things that need to be checked are as follows:

i) ***Viability of the isolates:*** viability of the microbes is measured by counting live cells under microscope or by checking the viable colony count as described in previous chapter (Chapter-6)

ii) ***Cross contamination of the isolates:*** Cross contamination can be checked by streaking or spreading the culture on nutrient agar plate.

After incubation for 24 hours colony characters are studied to check for presence of mixed population due to contamination.

iii) ***Any genetic modification:*** Genetic modification can be checked by PCR techniques where gene specific and species-specific primers are used to amplify a few set of marker genes. Amplification products are purified and sequenced by Sanger sequencing to check for any mutation.

iv) If the viability of the isolates is above 90% and they are free from contamination and genetic modification they can be used for experimental studies.

Chapter 8

Microbial Colony Characteristics

Microbes grow on solid media in the form of colonies. A colony can be defined as a visible mass of microbes originating from a single cell. They are homogenous and genetically identical population. Each microbe has a typical morphological character associated with the colony on the basis of which they can be visually identified.

On solid medium the following colony characters are observed:

1. Shape: Circular, irregular, radiate or rhizoid.

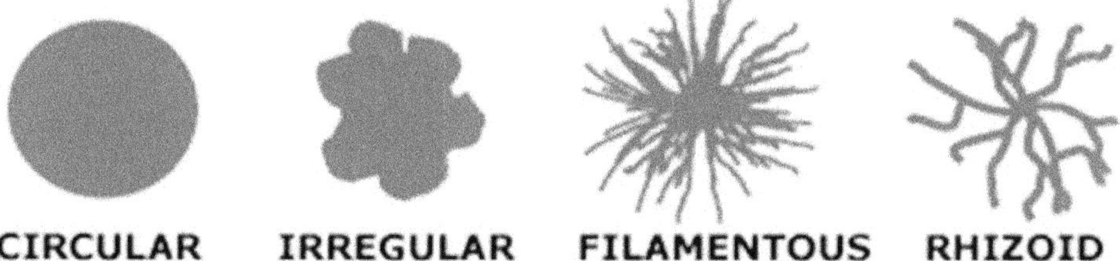

Fig. 8.1: The figure depicts the shape of colony.

2. Size: The size of the colony can be a useful characteristic for identification. The diameter of a representative colony may be measured.
3. Margin: Entire, wavy, lobate, filiform.

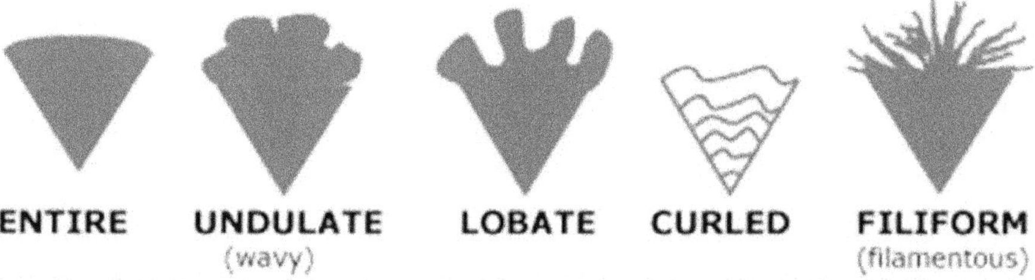

Fig. 8.2: The figure depicts the margin of the colony.

Elevation

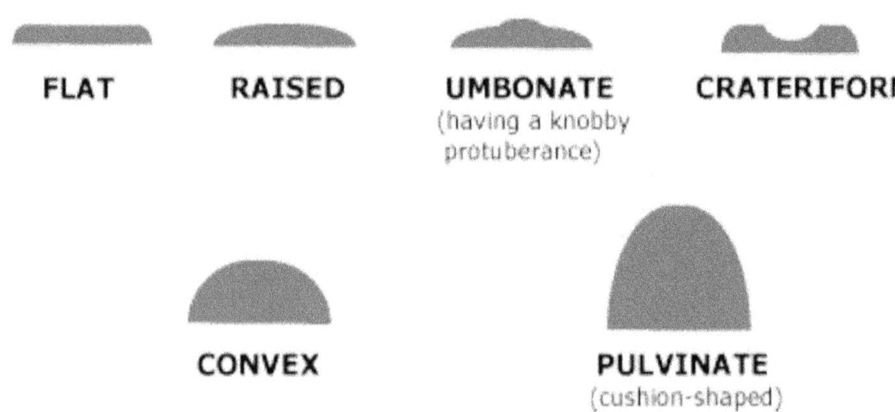

Fig. 8.3: The figure depicts the elevation of the colony.

4. Surface: Smooth, wavy, rough, granular, papillate, glistening etc.
5. Texture: Dry, moist, mucoid, brittle, viscous, butyrous etc.
6. Color: colorless or any visually distinct color.
7. Opacity of colony: transparent (clear), opaque (not transparent or clear), translucent (almost clear, but distorted vision–like looking through frosted glass), iridescent (changing colors in reflected light).

Chapter 9

Microscopic Observation

Gram's Staining

Principle

Gram staining is a method that differentiates bacteria in two large group- Gram positive and Gram negative. This method was discovered by Danish scientist and physician Hans Christian Joachim Gram in 1884. This method differentiates bacteria by the specific character of their cell walls. Gram positive bacteria have a thick network of peptidoglycan which is cross linked to transpeptidase enzyme which increases its rigidity, whereas Gram-negative bacteria have a thinner layer of peptidoglycan. This rigid peptidoglycan layer traps the Crystal Violet-Iodine complex and imparts purple colour to the cells. Crystal violet in aqueous environment dissociates into CV^+ and Cl^- ions which can easily enter the wall and membrane of both Gram-positive and Gram-negative cells. The CV^+ interacts with negatively charged components of bacterial cells thereby staining them purple. This is followed by addition of iodine which interacts with CV^+ to form large crystal violet iodine (CV-I) complexes. Ethanol which is used as decolorizing agent interacts with the lipids of the membranes of both Gram-positive and Gram negative bacteria and removes the outer membrane of the Gram-negative cell which is composed of lipopolysaccharide layer thereby making the Gram-negative cells walls leaky. The large CV-I complex leaks out of the thin peptidoglycan layer, whereas cross linked multilayered peptidoglycan of the Gram-positive cell gets dehydrated by the addition of ethanol and traps the large CV-I complexes within the cell.

After decolourization, the Gram-positive cell remains purple in colour, whereas the Gram-negative cell loses the purple colour which could then be visualized by safranin that is used to counter stain the cells.

Materials Required:

1. Clean glass slides
2. Inoculating loop
3. Spirit Lamp
4. Distilled water

5. Microbial cultures
6. Primary Stain - Crystal Violet
7. Mordant - Grams Iodine
8. Decolourizer - Ethyl Alcohol
9. Counter Stain - Safranin
10. Microscope

Method

24 hour grown bacterial cultures are used for Gram's staining purpose. A single colony is mixed with distilled water until it turns slightly turbid. Bacterial smear are prepared on a clean glass slide using an inoculating loop. The smear is heat fixed using spirit lamp and allowed to cool at room temperature for few minutes. Crystal Violet solution is added to the bacterial smear and incubated for 1 minute followed by washing with distilled water. The slide is then flooded with gram's iodine and incubated for 1 minute followed by washing with distilled water. Next, few drops of decolourizer was added onto the smear and incubated for 30 second followed by washing. Finally counter stain (safranin) is added and incubated for 1 minute, rinsed with distilled water and allowed to air dry. The slide is then observed under the light microscope.

Result

Color Of The Bacterial Cell	Grams's Reaction
Blue/Purple	Gram Positive
Red/Pink	Gram Negative

Acid Fast Stain (Ziehl-Neelsen Technique)

Principle

There are few organisms with wax-like cell walls composed of mycolic acid and fatty acids which make them impermeable. This character makes them highly resistant to disinfectants and dry conditions. These group of organisms are categorized as Acid Fast organisms. This techniques was first developed by Ziehl and later on modified by Neelsen. So this method is also called Ziehl-Neelsen staining technique. This method is specifically used for strains that could not be stained with Gram's stain.

Carbol fuchsin being lipid soluble, easily penetrates the cell wall upon heat fixing the cells leading to further penetration through lipid layer. This imparts red colour to the cells. A decolorizing agent made of 3% HCl prepared in 95% alcohol destains the non acid fast strains but cannot penetrate the lipid layer. Methylene blue which is used as counter stain when applied after decolourization step stains all the non acid fast cell that have lost the red colour. Therefore they appear blue while acid-fast cells retain the red colour.

Materials Required

11. Clean glass slides
12. Inoculating loop
13. Spirit Lamp
14. Distilled water
15. Microbial cultures
16. Primary Stain - Carbol fuchsin
17. Decolourizer - 3% HCl prepared in 95% alcohol
18. Counter Stain - Methylene Blue
19. Microscope

Method

A bacterial smear is prepared on a clean glass slide using inoculation loop. The smear is air dried and then heat fixed over a spirit lamp. The smear is stained with carbol fuchsin stain. The slide is heated to nearly 60°C and incubated for 5 minutes followed by washing with distilled water. Next the decolorizer is applied over the smear and incubated for 5 minutes or until the smear is sufficiently decolorized, i.e. pale pink. This is again followed by washing with distilled water. Methylene blue is now applied to counter stain the cells, incubated for 1-2 min followed by washing with distilled water. Finally the smear is air dried and examined microscopically.

Result:

Color Of The Bacterial Cell	Acid Fast Reaction
Red/Pink	Positive
Blue	Negative

Acridine Orange Stain

Principle

Acridine Orange is a fluorochrome stain that can be directly used to detect microorganisms in clinical samples. It easily permeates inside cells and specifically binds to nucleic acids. The advantage of this stain is that at low pH it differentially fluoresces on binding to the infecting microbe and the human cells. While the human cells and tissue material appear as pale green to yellow, bacteria fluoresce a bright orange at a pH of 3.5 - 4.0, thereby distinguishing both.

Materials Required

1. Clean glass slides
2. Inoculating loop
3. Spirit Lamp
4. Distilled water
5. Microbial cultures

6. Acridine orange
7. Glacial Acetic acid
8. Microscope

Method

A bacterial smear was prepared on a clean dry grease free glass slide and air dried. The slides are heat fixed with absolute methanol for 2 minutes. Next the slides are flooded with Acridine Orange and incubated for 2 minutes. This is followed by rinsing with distilled water and allowed to air dry. Finally the slide is observed under fluorescence microscope.

Result

Color Of The Bacterial Cell	Acid Fast Reaction
Orange	Bacteria
Pale Green	Human cells or tissue

Auramine-Rhodamine Technique

Principle

This technique is also known as Truant method for acid-fast staining. It is a fluorescent based method for detecting Acid Fast Bacilli. The acid fast bacteria are characterised by thick wall composed of waxes, lipids and Mycolic acid. The fluorochrome dye, Auramine-Rhodamine binds to the mycolic acid and forms a complex. This complex is resistant to acid alcohol. The counter stain potassium permanganate stains the non-acid fast strains and prevents nonspecific fluorescence.

Materials Required

1. Clean glass slides
2. Inoculating loop
3. Spirit Lamp
4. Distilled water
5. Microbial cultures
6. Primary Stain - Auramine Rhodamine
7. Decolourizer - 0.5 ml of conc.HCl in 100 ml of 70% ethanol.
8. Counter Stain - Potassium Permanganate
9. Microscope

Method

A thin smear of the bacterial culture is prepared on a glass slide and heat fixed using a spirit lamp. The slide is heated to 65-75 °C. Auramine O-Rhodamine B solution is applied to the slides and allowed to stain for 15 minutes. This is followed by washing with distilled water. The smear is flooded with decolorizing agent for 2 to 3 minutes and again washed with distilled water. All the excess water is removed and the slides are treated with counter stain and incubate for 2 minutes. Time is critical during counterstaining because excess potassium permanganate may quench fluorescence of acid-fast bacilli. The slides are rinsed and air dried and finally observed under fluorescent microscope.

Calcofluor White Staining

Principle

Calcofluor is a specific stain for β-glucans and chitin. It is a fluorescent stain for rapid detection of fungus. The dye fluoresces as it is exposed to ultraviolet light.

Materials Required

1. Solution A- Potassium hydroxide reagent.

   Potassium hydroxide (10%), Glycerin (10%), Water

2. Solution B- Calcofluor white reagent.

   Calcofluor white powder (0.1%) in the distilled water

Method

A clean grease free slide is taken, on which one drop of each solution A and B is placed at the centre slide and mixed. The isolate is placed on the solution and a clean cover slip is placed over the sample. It is slightly pressed and the excess liquid is wiped off. The slide is slightly warmed under a spirit lamp and examined microscopically.

Result

Calcofluor white stain shows absorption peak at 347-nm which is under ultraviolet range. Under this condition the fungal filaments fluoresce bright apple green in color.

Capsule Stain

Principle

This is a differential stain which selectively stains external Capsules surrounding bacterial cells. Capsules are a protective layer secreted by the bacterium outside the cell wall which is basically composed of polysaccharides. Capsulated bacteria are generally virulent as the capsule layer prevents them from desiccation, phagocytosis as well as detergents. Since capsule layers are non-ionic and would not bind to any acidic or basic stains, therefore the strategy is to do a double staining i.e. the background is stained with acidic stain and the cell is stained with basic stain.

Materials Required

Cell Stain: Crystal Violet (1%)

Background Stain: India Ink, Nigrosin (10%), copper sulphate (20%)

Method

In case when India Ink, Nigrosin or Congo Red is used, first a drop of any of these dye is placed on a clean grease free glass slide. The bacterial sample is placed over the dye and a clean smear is prepared using another glass slide. The slide is air dried and crystal violet is flooded over the slide. Excess crystal violet dye is removed by placing the slide in a tilted position. The smear is air dried and visualized under microscope.

When Copper sulphate is used as background stain, first the cells are stained with crystal violet as mentioned above. Excess crystal violet is removed by tilting the slide. It is air dried followed by addition of copper sulphate (20%). The slide is air dried and observed under microscope.

Result

In the first case when India ink, Nigrosin or Congo red is used, they stain the background while the Crystal violet stains the cells. When the cells are visualized under microscope, the capsule appears as a halo around the purple cells over a dark background.

In the second case, when copper sulphate in used cells appear purple and the capsule appears light blue. The copper sulphate solution acts as the decolorizing agent as well as counter stain. It decolorizes the capsule and simultaneously counter stains the capsule. As a result the capsule appears as a faint blue halo around a purple cell.

Endospore Stain

Principle

Vegetative cells under stress conditions enter a metabolically inactive and dormant stage called endospores. These resistant structures protect the cells during unfavourable conditions. This staining method is used to differentiate endospores from vegetative cells. Since the spores have a resistant wall they retain the primary stain which is forced into the cells by heating the samples, whereas the vegetative cells loose the primary stain as their cell membrane gets ruptured during heat fixing and they only retain counter stain.

Materials Required

1. Clean glass slides
2. Inoculating loop
3. Spirit Lamp
4. Microbial cultures
5. Primary Stain: Malachite green (0.5% (wt/vol) aqueous solution)
6. Distilled Water as decolorizing agent
7. Counter Stain: Safranin (2.5% (wt/vol) alcoholic solution)
8. Microscope

Method

A clean grease free slide is taken and bacterial smear is prepared in a sterile condition. The smear is air dried and heat fixed and covered with a blotting paper which uniformly covers the slide. Malachite green stain solution is added over the blotting paper so that is saturated enough to keep the smear moist. The stained smear is heated over lamp for 5 minutes. During warming the smear is kept moist by addition of staining solution as per requirements. After heating the slide is washed with tap water and counterstained with safranin for 30 seconds. Finally the slide is again washed with tap water and air dried. The slide is examined under microscope to detect endospores.

Result

Endospores will appear as bright green and the vegetative cells get counterstained with safranin and appear as red or pink.

Flagella Stain

Principle

Flagella are locomotory organs of microbes. Since they have a very fine structure it is difficult to observe them under microscope. So in flagella staining technique the basic principle employed is to add stains that increase the thickness of the flagella, so that they could be observed under microscope.

Materials Required

1. Clean glass slides
2. Inoculating loop
3. Microbial cultures
4. Primary Stain: Leifson's stain
5. Distilled Water
6. 1 % methylene blue
7. Microscope

Method

A loopful of bacteria from agar slant is suspended in 2 ml distilled water and the suspension is allowed to incubate for 1hour. A smear from the bacterial suspension is prepared on clean, grease free slide. The slide is kept in slant position while preparing smear. The smear is air dried before staining. The staining solution is added drop wise till a thin shiny film of the stain is observed. The smear is washed gently with water and treated with 1 % methylene blue for 1 minute. Finally the smear is washed with water, air dried and observed under microscope.

Result

The flagella appear red in colour and bacterial cell appear blue.

Lactophenol Cotton Blue (LPCB) Wet Mount

Principle

This staining method is specifically used for fungus. As the name of stain indicates, the stain comprises of phenol, lactic acid and cotton blue stain. The phenol kills all living organisms, lactic acid helps in preserving fungal structures and cotton blue stains chitin present in fungal cell wall.

Materials Required

1. Clean glass slides
2. Inoculating wire
3. Fungal cultures
4. Lactophenol cotton blue dye
5. 70% Ethanol
6. Microscope

Method

Few drops of 70% ethanol placed on a clean and grease free slide. Fungal filaments or hyphae are carefully removed from slant and placed on the ethanol drop. Spread the sample smoothly using a fine needle. Add lactophenol cotton blue dye to the immersed samples and carefully place cover slip avoiding air bubbles. The mount can now be observed under microscope.

Result

Fungal elements appear intense blue under microscope.

Sudan B Staining

Principle

Sudan Black B is a nonfluorescent, thermostable fat-soluble diazo dye used for staining of neutral triglycerides and lipids. Since it is insoluble in water but dissolves in fat, therefore this dye will accumulate in fat globules within a cell.

Materials Required

1. 3% Sudan Black B stain prepared in 60% Ethanol
2. 0.5%(w/v) safranine in water
3. Glass slide
4. Microscope

Method

1. Prepare a smear of the bacteria
2. Allow the smear to dry and heat fix
3. Flood dried fixed smear with Sudan black B stain
4. Incubate for 10 minutes
5. Drain off the excess dye
6. Blot dry
7. Apply safranine for 10-15 seconds
8. Rinse with tap water
9. Air dry

10. Observe stained smear under the oil immersion objective

Result

Globules of fat appear blue-black within the red cytoplasm.

Albert's Staining For *C. Diphtheriae*

Principle

C. diphtheriae is Gram-positive, aerobic, nonmotile, toxin-producing, club-shaped bacillus bacteria. A typical feature is the presence of numerous metachromatic granules that give the bacillus beaded or barred appearance.

Materials Required

1. Albert stain I

   Toluidine blue 0.15 gm

   Malachite green 0.20 gm

   Glacial acetic acid 1.0 ml

   Alcohol(95%) 2.0 ml

   Distilled water 100 ml

2. Albert stain II

   Iodine 2.0 gm

   Potassium iodide 3.0 gm

   Distilled water 300 ml

Method

1. Heat fix the bacterial smear.
2. Flood the heat-fixed smear with Albert stain I. Incubate for 2 minutes.
3. Rinse with water.
4. Flood the smear with Albert stain II. Incubate for 2 minutes.
5. Rinse with water, blot dry and observe.

Result

These granules appear bluish black whereas the body of bacilli appear green or bluish green.

Giemsa Stain

Principle

Giemsa stain is used to differentiate nuclear and/or cytoplasmic morphology of platelets, RBCs, WBCs, and parasites. It differentially stains human and bacterial cells. It can be used for histopathological diagnosis of malaria and some other spirochete and protozoan blood parasites.

Materials Required

1. Giemsa Stain

2. 100% Methanol
3. Glass slide
4. Microscope

Method

1. Prepare a thin smear of blood.
2. Fix the smear by addition of 100% methanol for 30 seconds.
3. Flood the stain slowly on the slide until the blood smear is completely covered.
4. Incubate for 10 minutes.
5. Discard the excess stain from the slide and gently rinse with distilled water.
6. Allow the slides to air-dry and observe under microscope.

Result

Giemsa solution is composed of eosin and methylene blue (azure). The eosin component stains the parasite nucleus red, while the methylene blue component stains the cytoplasm blue.

Lugol's Iodine Stain

Principle

Lugol's iodine is a non- specific, rapid contrast dye used for differentiating intestinal protozoa and helminths ova or larvae from host WBC. The organisms take up dye that stains the protozoan nuclei and intra cytoplasmic organelles brown while other objects in the sample remain colorless.

Materials Required

1. Lugol's Iodine solution
2. Faecal sample
3. PBS
4. Microscope

Method

1. Dissolve the faecal sample in PBS and prepare a thin smear of faecal sample.
2. Dilute Lugol's iodine 1:5 with sterile de-ionized water and flood over the wet mount.
3. Place a coverslip on the stained mount and observe under microscope.

Result

The parasite appears brown colour while other components appear colourless.

Chapter 10

Biochemical Characterization

Triple Sugar Iron Test (TSI)

Principle

The Triple Sugar Iron test is a microbiological test named for its ability to test microorganisms' ability to ferment sugars and to produce hydrogen sulfide. The TSI slant is a test tube that contains agar, a pH-sensitive dye (phenol red), 1% lactose, 1% sucrose, 0.1% glucose as well as sodium thiosulfate and ferrous sulfate. Fermentation of these sugars and production of sulphide leads to color change of the slant (Hajna, 1945).

Materials Required

1. Bacterial Culture
2. TSI Medium (Beef extract 3g/l, Peptone 2g/l, Yeast extract 3g/l, Lactose 1g/l, Sucrose 1g/l, Dextrose monohydrate 1g/l, Ferrous sulphate 0.2g/l, Sodium chloride 5g/l, Sodium thiosulphate 0.3g/l, Phenol red 0.024g/l, Agar 12g/l)
3. Incubator

Method

Slants were prepared using TSI agar medium in culture tube. After solidification of the slant, a single colony from the pure culture is streaked on the slant and allowed to incubate at the optimum temperature required for the microbe. After 24 hours of incubation, the culture tubes are taken out of the incubator and the colour change in the slant is noted down.

Result

Results (slant/butt)	Symbol	Interpretation
Red/yellow	K/A	Glucose fermentation only; Peptone catabolised
Yellow/yellow	A/A	Glucose and lactose and/or sucrose fermentation
Red/red	K/K	No fermentation; Peptone catabolised
Red/no color change	K/NC	No fermentation; Peptone used aerobically
Yellow/yellow with bubbles	A/A,G	Glucose and lactose and/or sucrose fermentation; Gas produced
Red/yellow with bubbles	K/A,G	Glucose fermentation only; Gas produced

Red/yellow with bubbles and black precipitate	K/A,G, H_2S	Glucose fermentation only; Gas produced; H_2S produced
Red/yellow with black precipitate	K/A, H_2S	Glucose fermentation only; H_2S produced
Yellow/yellow with black precipitate	A/A, H_2S	Glucose and lactose and/or sucrose fermentation; H_2S produced
No change/no change	NC/NC	No fermentation

A=acid production; K=alkaline reaction; G=gas production; H_2S=sulfur reduction

Citrate Utilization Test

Principle

The citrate utilization test notices the capability of an organism to consume citrate as the sole source of carbon and energy for growth and metabolism. The principle is based on the breaking down of citrate to oxaloacetate and acetate. Bacteria are inoculated on a medium containing sodium citrate and a pH indicator such as bromothymol blue. This medium also comprises inorganic ammonium salts, which are utilized as nitrogen source. Bacteria decompose the citrate in the presence of enzyme citrate lyase which breaks down citrate to oxaloacetate and acetate. Oxaloacetate is further decomposed in to pyruvate and carbon dioxide (CO_2). Production of sodium bicarbonate ($NaHCO_3$) as well as ammonia (NH_3) from the use of sodium citrate and ammonium salts results in alkaline pH. This results in a change of the medium's color from green to blue (Simmons, 1926).

Materials Required

1. Bacterial Culture
2. Simmon's citrate agar medium (sodium chloride 5.0gm, sodium citrate (dehydrate) 2.0 gm, Number and unit ammonium dihydrogen phosphate 1.0 gm, dipotassium phosphate 1.0 gm, magnesium sulfate (heptahydrate) 0.2 gm). 24.28 grams of the media was suspended in 1000 ml distilled water, mix well and sterilize by autoclaving.
3. Incubator

Method

Slants were prepared using Simmon's citrate agar medium in culture tube. After solidification of the slant, a single colony from the pure culture is streaked on the slant and allowed to incubate at the optimum, temperature required for the microbe. After 24 hours of incubation, the culture tubes are taken out of the incubator and the colour change in the slant is noted down.

Result

Citrate positive:	Growth is observed on the slant as well as the slant appears intense blue. The alkaline by-products produced during breakdown of sodium citrate led to increase in pH of the medium (around 7.6) which results in change in colour of green to blue.
Citrate negative	No growth or colour change of the stab is observed.

Mannitol Utilization & Motility Test

Principle

Mannitol motility medium is a bacterial growth medium used to detect the ability of bacteria to ferment mannitol and produce nitrogen gas. When inoculated with a sample organism and allowed to incubate, the medium will change color from red to yellow to indicate that the mannitol has been fermented. The pattern of color change indicates the motility of the organism.

Materials Required

1. Bacterial Culture
2. Mannitol motility agar medium (peptic digest of animal tissue 20g/l, mannitol 2g/l, potassium nitrate 1g/l, phenol red 0.04g/l, agar 3g/l, Final pH (at 25°C) 7.6±0.2)

   26.04 grams of the media was suspended in 1000 ml distilled water, mix well and sterilize by autoclaving. The agar stab is kept in an upright position.
3. Incubator

Method

Slants were prepared using Mannitol motility agar medium in culture tube. After solidification of the slant, a single colony from the pure culture is streaked on the slant and allowed to incubate at the optimum temperature required for the microbe. After 24 hours of incubation, the culture tubes are taken out of the incubator and the colour change in the slant is noted down.

Result

Mannitol utilization positive	**Stab turns yellow at pH<6.8**
Mannitol utilization negative	Stab turns pink at pH>8.4
Motile	Diffused growth leading to change in color of stab
Non-motile	Growth confined to stab line with uniform margin

Nitrate Reduction Test

Principle

This test is performed to check the ability of microbes to produce nitrate reductase enzyme that hydrolyze nitrate (NO_3^-) to nitrite (NO_2^-). Also this is a characteristic test to distinguish Enterobactericae member.

The nitrate reductase present in the microbe converts nitrate to nitrite and the nitrite converts to nitrous acid in the media. Addition of sulfanilic acid leads to reaction with nitrous acid to produce diazotized sulfanilic acid. This subsequently reacts with alpha-naphthylamine to form a red-coloured precipitate which turns the media red. This is a positive result for nitrate reduction. A negative result may have two consequences, either the microbe does not have the nitrate reductase to convert nitrate to nitrite or the microbe denitrifies the nitrate or nitrite to produce ammonia or molecular nitrogen. Such condition is cross confirmed by addition of zinc powder. A change in colour of tube into red means nitrate is present in unreduced condition. Therefore, a red coloured on the second step is a negative result. Zinc reduces the nitrate to nitrite, and the nitrite forms nitrous acid, which reacts with sulfanilic acid. The diazotized sulfanilic acid that was thereby produced reacts with the alpha-naphthylamine to create the red colour compound. If no red colour forms after addition of zinc, it can be concluded that no residual nitrate is present and all the nitrate have been denitrified to produce ammonia or molecular nitrogen.

Materials Required

1. Bacterial culture
2. Nitrate broth
3. Sulphalinic acid reagent, alpha napthylamine reagent, zinc dust

Method

Nitrate broth is inoculated with healthy growing cells. It is incubated at an appropriate temperature for 24 to 48 hours. 1ml each of sulfanilic acid and alpha-naphthylamine is added to the overnight grown cultures. A change in colour to red indicates a positive nitrate reduction test. If no colour appears, small amount of zinc is added to the culture. At this point, a colour change to red indicates a negative nitrate reduction test

Result

Red after addition of sulphalinic acid reagent, alpha napthylamine reagent	Presence of nitrate reductase
Red after addition of zinc	Absence of nitrate reductase
No colour after addition of zinc	Denitrification of nitrate

Gelatin Hydrolysis Test

Principle

This test is used to determine the ability of an organism to produce extracellular proteolytic enzyme, gelatinases that hydrolyze gelatin. The presence of gelatinases is detected using a nutrient gelatin medium. This medium is a simple medium composed of gelatin peptone and beef extract. When nutrient gelatin tube is inoculated with gelatinases positive organisms, the secreted gelatinases will liquefy the gelatin, resulting in the liquefaction of the medium. While the gelatinase negative organism don't secret enzymes and thus liquefaction of media does not occur.

Materials Required

1. Bacterial culture
2. Nutrient gelatin medium (Nutrient broth 13g/l, gelatin 120g/l)
3. Incubator

Method

Stabs prepared from nutrient gelatin medium were inoculated with healthy growing cells. It is incubated at an appropriate temperature for 24 hours. Post incubation, the stab is tested for the consistency of the medium.

Result

Gelatinase positive	Stab liquefies
Gelatinase negative	Stab remains solidified

Urease Production

Principle

Few enteric bacteria produce an exozyme urease, which breaks down urea into carbon dioxide and ammonia. The ammonia combines with carbon dioxide and water to form ammonium carbonate. Ammonium carbonate turns the medium alkaline, which lead to change in colour of pH indicator phenol red from orange yellow to bright pink. This test is perform to identify microbes causing urinary tract infection and more specifically used to differentiate members of the *genus Proteus*.

Materials Required

1. Bacterial culture
2. Nutrient broth (pH 6.8-7.0)
3. Urea (20g/l)
4. Phenol red (0.01g/l)
5. Incubator

Method

Urea broth is prepared by dissolving appropriate amounts of phenol red to nutrient broth. The media is sterilized by autoclaving. It is allowed to cool and urea which is filter sterilized is added after the media cools down to room temperature. The medium is inoculated with healthy growing cells. It is incubated at an appropriate temperature for 24 hours. Post incubation, the stab is tested for the colour change of the medium.

Result

Yellow to pink	Positive If colour change appears within 1-2 hours organisms are rapid urease-positive
No colour change	Negative

Oxidase Activity Test

Principle

The test is performed to detect the presence cytochrome oxidase enzyme which oxidises cytochrome c. These enzymes catalyse the transport of electrons from donor compounds to electron acceptors. In this test the coloured reagent used is N,N,N′,N′-tetramethyl-p-phenylenediamine dihydrochloride which gets oxidized by cytochrome oxidase and changes colour to blue or purple.

Materials Required

1. Bacteria culture
2. Oxidase disc (Filter papers impregnated with the dye)

Method

Oxidase disc can be directly procured or prepared in lab by adding few drops of N, N, N′, N′-tetramethyl-p-phenylenediamine dihydrochloride reagent to a filter paper. It is allowed to dry for few minutes and then fresh bacterial colonies picked using a wooden loop or needle and streaked on the disc.

Result

Colour changes to blue to purple in 10-20 seconds	Positive
No colour change	Negative
Colour change after 30 second	False positive. Change in colour due to oxidation of dye by overexposure of the strip in air.

Indole Production

Principle

The various enzymes involved in the degradation of tryptophan to indole are collectively called as tryptophanase, a general term used to denote the complete system of enzymes. The presence of indole is detected by the Kovac's reagent strip which turns pink in the presence of indole. This test is performed to differentiate Enterobacteriaceae from other genera.

Materials Required

1. Bacteria culture
2. Nutrient broth
3. Kovac's reagent strip
4. Incubator

Method

Kovac's reagent strips are sterile filter paper strips impregnated with Kovac's reagent. Indole production by organisms is observed by inserting the Kovac's reagent strip between the plug and inner wall of the tube and incubating at 35-37°C for 18-24 hours.

Result

Strip turns pink	Positive for tryptophanase
No colour change	Negative for tryptophanase

Coagulase Test

Principle

Coagulase is the enzyme involved in the conversion of fibrinogen to fibrin. This test is performed to differentiate pathogenic and non-pathogenic members of *Staphylococcus*. Coagulase is present in bound as well as in free form. Bound coagulase remains attached to the bacterial cell membrane and directly reacts with fibrinogen and leads to clumping of bacterial cells, whereas free coagulase is secreted by the bacteria which reacts with coagulase reacting factor (CRF) present in plasma and forms thrombin. This converts fibrinogen to fibrin resulting in clotting of plasma.

Materials Required

1. Bacterial culture
2. Plasma (rabbit/human)

Method

There are two methods for performing this test. The slide test is performed to detect bound coagulase and the tube method is done to test the presence of free coagulase.

Slide test

A clean grease free slide is taken. A drop of water is placed on the slide and a colony from the pure culture is dissolved in this water droplet. To this bacterial suspension, a drop of plasma is added and mixed smoothly. Then check for clumping within 10sec.

Tube test

Plasma is diluted in commercially available saline (0.9% NaCl) in 1:10 ratio. 1 ml of diluted plasma is taken in clean test tube. To the diluted plasma, should be 100μ of overnight grown culture is added. It is incubated for 4hours and clumping is observed.

Result

Slide Test: Clumping within 10sec	Positive for bound coagulase
Slide Test: Clumping after 10sec	Perform tube test to confirm presence of free coagulase
Tube test: Clumping	Positive for free coagulase

Hemolysin Test

Principle

This test is performed to analyze the ability of bacteria to lyse red blood cells. Blood agar media is used to perform this test.

Materials Required

1. Bacterial culture
2. Blood agar plate

Method

An isolated colony is picked using a sterile inoculating loop and streaked on a blood agar plate. The plate is incubated for 24–48 h. Post incubation any presence of a zone of clearing or discoloration around isolated colonies is observed.

Result

Bacteria that can completely lyse the blood cells, causing a clearing around the colony, are called β-*hemolytic bacteria*. Bacteria that can partially break down the blood cells, causing a green or brown discoloration of the agar around the colony, are called α-*hemolytic bacteria*. Bacteria that cannot lyse the cells, causing no change in the agar, are called γ-*hemolytic*.

Bile Esculin Agar Test

Principle

This test is performed to isolate and identify group D streptococci and enterococci bacteria that have the ability to hydrolyze esculin in the presence of bile.

The media comprises of esculin, peptone and bile. While esculin and peptone are source of nutrition for the bacteria, bile acts as an inhibitor for the growth of Gram-positive bacteria other than group D streptococci and enterococci. Ferric citrate is used as a color indicator.

Esculin is a glycoside, which could be hydrolyzed by manybacteria, but few can do so in the presence of bile.

The free esculetin released after hydrolysis of esculin, reacts with ferric citrate to form a phenolic iron complex, which turns the agar slant dark brown.

Materials Required

1. Bacterial culture
2. Bile esculin agar (the media is prepared as per manufacturer's instruction)

Method

Slants are prepared using Bile esculin agar base. They are inoculated with a single colony isolated from pure culture. Slants are incubated for 24-48 hours and observed for change in colour.

Result

An agar slant that is more than half darkened after 48 hours incubation	Bile-esculin positive
If the slant has darkened less than half	Negative

Spirit Blue Agar Test

Principle

Spirit blue agar is used for detection of lipase producing microbes. Some group of bacteria use lipid as carbon source to generate energy. They have lipase enzyme that is capable of breaking down lipids. Spirit blue agar is an emulsion of lipids like olive oil and spirit blue.

Materials Required

1. Microbial cultures
2. Spirit blue agar plates

Method:

1. Prepare spirit blue agar plate by suspending 32.15 gm of spirit blue agar powder in 1000ml distilled water. Sterilize by autoclaving and pour it in sterile Petri dishes and allow to solidify.
2. Streak the microbial culture on the plate and incubate at appropriate temperature.
3. After growth of microbe on the plate, observe for change around the colony.

Result:

The medium normally appears opaque and light blue in color. Colonies of lipolytic organisms develop a clear zone and /or a deep blue color around the colony.

10.13 Starch Hydrolysis Test

Principle:

Some group of bacteria possess enzymes alpha-amylase and oligo-1,6-glucosidase that can hydrolyze starch (amylose and amylopectin). Since these are long chain oligosaccharides, some microbes cannot uptake them through cell wall. They therefore secrete alpha-amylase and oligo-1, 6-glucosidase enzymes to extracellular medium which breaks these complex oligosaccharides to simple glucose units. This glucose can then be readily uptaken by the microbe as a carbon source. Iodine is used as a staining agent to detect hydrolysis of starch.

Materials Required:

1. Starch agar (nutrient agar medium to which starch is added)
2. Microbial culture
3. Grams iodine

Method

1. Prepare a starch agar plate by adding 0.2-0.5% soluble starch to nutrient agar media. Mix uniformly and sterilize by auoclaving. Pour the sterilized media into Petri dishes and allow to solidify.
2. Streak the colonies on starch agar plate and allow to incubate at appropriate temperature.
3. After the growth of microbe on starch agar plate, stain it with Gram's iodine and observe for change in the plate.

Result

The iodine reacts with the starch to form a dark brown colour. Thus, hydrolysis of the starch will create a clear zone around the bacterial growth.

Methyl Red / Voges-Proskauer (MR/VP)

Principle

This test is performed to detect mixed acid fermentative pathway of the microbe. Some microbe utilize glucose and produce acetic acid, lactic acid, formic acid and ethanol through mixed acid fermentation pathway. The type of acid produced varies from species to species. Whatever acid may be formed, it accumulates in the media and turns methyl red indicator from yellow to red.

Some other microbe have an active 2,3 butanediol fermentation pathway which ferment glucose and produce a 2,3 butanediol end product instead of organic acids. The Voges-Proskauer test detects the presence of acetoin, a precursor of 2,3 butanediol.

Materials Required

1. MRVP broth (pH 6.9)
2. 0.02%Methyl red solution prepared in 95% ethanol
3. 5% α-naphthol
4. 40% KOH
5. Microbial culture

Method

MR Test

1. Prepare MRVP media as per manufacturer's instruction.
2. Inoculate the media with 1% overnight grown pre-culture.
3. Incubate aerobically at 37°C for 24 hours.
4. Aliquot 1ml of the culture to a clean test tube and add 2 to 3 drops of methyl red indicator. Observe for change in colour immediately.

VP Test

1. Aliquot 1ml of the above mentioned culture to a clean test tube and add 0.6 ml of 5% α-naphthol, followed by 0.2 ml of 40% KOH (follow the order of addition of reagents).
2. The culture is shaken vigorously and set aside for about one hour until the results can be read.

Result

MR Test

A distinct red colour indicates a positive result (MR+) and no change or yellow colour indicates negative result (MR-)

VP Test

If the culture is positive for acetoin, it will turn "brownish-red to pink" (VP+). If the culture is negative for acetoin, it will turn "brownish-green to yellow" (VP-). Vigorous shaking increases oxygen availability in the culture and in the presence of oxygen and 40% KOH, acetoin is converted to diacetyl.α-naphthol serves as a catalyst to bring out a red complex.

MacConkey Agar Test

Principle

MacConkey agar is used for the isolation of gram-negative enteric bacteria and for differentiation of lactose fermenting from lactose non-fermenting gram-negative bacteria. Presence of bile salts and crystal violet inhibit the growth of Gram positive organisms. Lactose fermentation is the basis of differentiation. Neutral red is used as pH indicator that turns red on acid formation (below pH 6.5) due to fermentation of lactose.

Materials Required

1. MacConkey agar
2. Microbial culture

Method

1. Prepare MacConkey agar plate as per manufacturer instruction.
2. Streak the microbial culture and allow the plate to incubate at appropriate temperature.
3. After the appearance of colonies on the plate observe for color change

Result

Lactose-fermenting organisms grow as pink to brick red colonies with or without a zone of precipitated bile. Non-lactose fermenting organisms grow as colourless or clear colonies

Hippurate Hydrolysis Test

Principle

Hippurate hydrolysis test is used in the presumptive identification of *Gardnerella vaginalis, Campylobacter jejuni, Listeria monocytogenes* and group B streptococci. In this assay the ability of microbe to hydrolyze hippuric acid to benzoic acid and glycine by enzyme hippuricase is tested. The glycine end product is detected by the addition of ninhydrin reagent.

Materials Required

1. Hippurate hydrolysis broth
2. Microbial culture
3. Ninhydrin reagent

Method

1. Prepare the hippurate hydrolysis broth as per manufacturer's instruction.
2. Inoculate the microbe into the sterile broth and incubate for 48 hours till dense growth is achieved.
3. Post incubation add 0.2 ml ninhydrin and again incubate at 37°C for 15-20 minutes and observe the change in colour.

Result

Development of a deep purple color within 15 minutes is a positive result. No change in colour within 15 minutes is a negative result.

Antibiotic Susceptibility Test

Principle

Antibiotics are drugs that inhibit the growth of microorganisms. There are several antibiotics that are naturally produced by microorganisms whereas various other antibiotics can be biochemically synthesized. Antibiotics are selectively toxic towards microorganisms, therefore while few microbes are resistant to them, other are susceptible. Also, the level of resistance and susceptibility differs among microbial population. Therefore in order to decide the most suitable drug for a pathogen, antibiotic susceptibility test is performed.

Two common experiments done to check the antibiotic susceptibility are disk diffusion method and serial dilution method.

Disk diffusion method

This method is a qualitative test which gives a broad idea whether the organism is resistant or susceptible. As the name suggests a disc soaked in the antibiotics is placed on a bacterial lawn. The antibiotic in the filter paper diffuses onto the nutrient agar plate and kills the microbes in the surrounding area, thereby creating a clearance zone. This area is called zone of inhibition. This diameter is measured and matched with standard values to check whether the organism is resistant or susceptible.

Materials Required

1. Nutrient agar plates
2. Antibiotics to be tested
3. Disc made up of filter paper
4. Forcep

Method

Filter paper disc are impregnated with the antibiotics that has to be tested. These filter papers are placed on a nutrient agar plate having a bacterial lawn. They are incubated at required temperature for 24 hours and post incubation zone of inhibition is measured.

Result

Measure the diameter of the Zone of Inhibition and compare it with standard values for the given antibiotic.

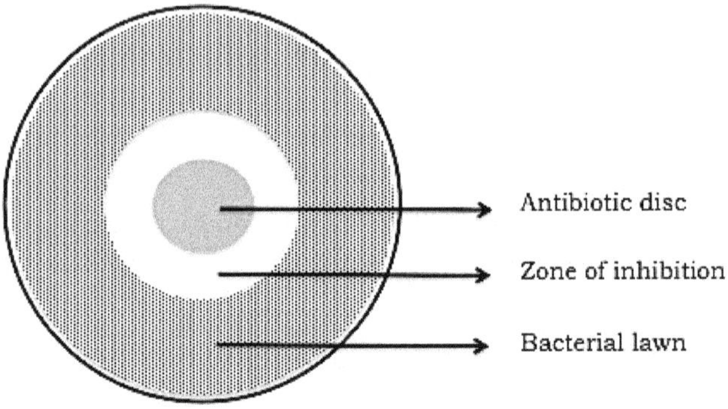

Antibiotic disc
Zone of inhibition
Bacterial lawn

Fig. 10.1: Schematic representation of Agar plate showing zone of inhibition produced by Antibiotic disc.

Serial Dilution Method

This is a quantitative

way of estimating the concentration of antibiotic required for growth inhibition. The minimum amount of antibiotic that restricts the growth of the microbe is termed as Minimum Inhibitory Concentration (MIC). This value differs for each antibiotic as well as different organism depending upon their susceptibility or resistance. MIC value is very crucial for prescribing the dose required for treatment of microbial infection. Similarly lethal dose can also be estimated from this method. Lethal dose (LD_{50}) is defined as the concentration at which half the population is dead.

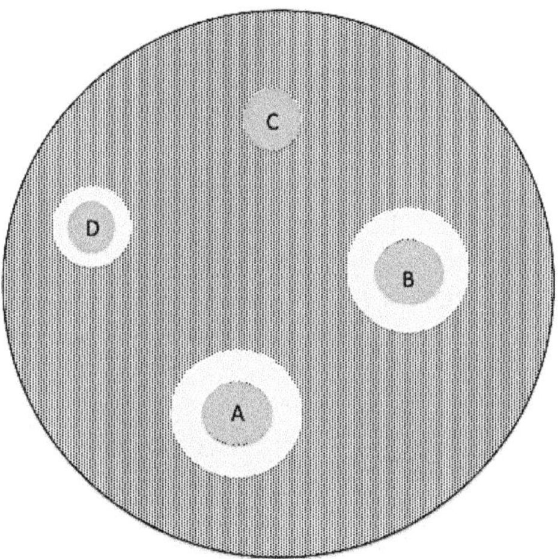

Fig. 10.2: Schematic representation of Agar plate showing differential zone of inhibition produced by different Antibiotic disc. Antibiotic A, B, D showing zone of inhibition (microbe is susceptible) whereas C has no zone of inhibition (microbe is resistant).

Materials Required

1. Nutrient broth
2. Antibiotics to be tested

Method

1ml of overnight grown microbial culture is taken in culture tubes, to which the antibiotic to be tested is serially diluted in the range of desired concentration gradient (eg: 32µl/ml, 16µl/ml, 8µl/ml, 4µl/ml, 2µl/ml, 1µl/ml). The tubes are incubated at desired temperature for 24 hours and post incubation the turbidity of the cultures is measured spectrophotometrically. A positive control is also set up simultaneously where an antibiotic showing growth inhibition is added.

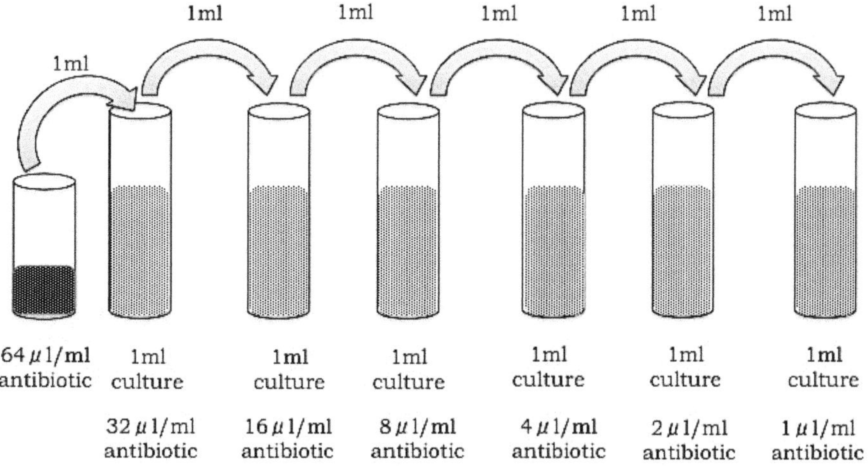

Fig. 10.3: Schematic representation of Serial dilution method to test Minimum Inhibitory Concentration (MIC).

Chapter 11

Molecular Characterization

Restriction Fragment Length Polymorphism (RFLP)

Principle

Restriction Fragment Length Polymorphism (RFLP) is a technique in which organisms may be differentiated on the basis of variation at DNA level. The principle of this analysis is to compare restriction digestion profiles of DNA samples isolated from different individuals. RFLP is used as a molecular marker where fragments of different lengths are generated after digestion of the DNA with specific restriction endonucleases. The homologous sequences having variations will generate a typical set of fragments with varying sizes. The resulting DNA fragments are then separated on the basis of their size and compared with related or unknown individuals (Narayanan, 1991).

Materials Required

1. DNA samples isolated from various organisms that have to be analyze
2. Restriction enzyme with compatible assay buffers
3. 1Kb DNA ladder
4. 0.8 % Agarose gel
5. 50X TAE buffer
6. EtBr for visualization
7. DNA loading dye (6X)
8. Gel documentation system with imager

Method

DNA isolation is the first critical step, where the method to be employed is designed on the basis of the quality and quantity of the purified DNA. Next Restriction digestion mixture (50µl) is prepared which comprises of the following components

DNA sample – 100 ng

10X assay buffer

Restriction enzyme- 1 unit

Molecular grade water

All the components are mixed well and incubated at recommended temperature for 2-3 hours. After incubation add 8µl of 6X loading dye and run the samples on 0.8% agarose gel alongside 1Kb DNA ladder. The number of restriction digestion mixture to be prepared depends on the number of samples to be analyzed. For each sample one set of mixture is prepared as per the given recipe.

Result

The figure is the pictorial representation of the DNA fragments obtained after restriction digestion followed by agarose gel electrophoresis of the samples. The restriction pattern of the samples is compared with the pattern obtained for reference sample. The organisms which are more related would produce very similar restriction patterns whereas unrelated organisms or homologous sequences having mutation would produce different restriction pattern.

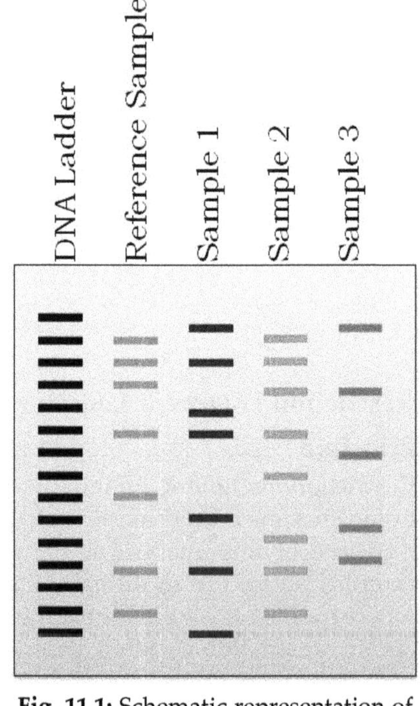

Fig. 11.1: Schematic representation of Agarose gels showing RFLP bands obtained from different DNA samples

Random Amplified Polymorphic DNA (RAPD)

Principle

RAPD is a PCR based technique used to analyze the DNA fingerprint of an individual. In this method random primers (6-10 bp) are designed which anneal to complementary sequences within the genomic DNA. If the random set of primers bind to sites which are in the range of 0.5-5KB then, amplified products are generated. Within a genomic DNA around 1-10 such priming sites may appear thereby producing discrete amplified bands of different sizes. These polymorphic bands are then used for comparison between two species (Williams, 1990).

Materials Required

Method

Step1: Preparation of master mix

- ◈ To prepare master mix for PCR, add the following items precisely.

  dNTP- 2mM

  Primer- 2mM

  10X Buffer- 1X

  Taq Polymerase- 1 unit

Molecular biology grade water- to be used to make up total volume.

- ◈ Aliquot 20µl of the master mix into the vials.
- ◈ Add 25-50ng of DNA isolated from different samples.

Step 2: Setting up PCR programme

Initial denaturation- 95°C, 2 min

(Denaturation- 95°C, 1min

Annealing- 35°C-40°C (can be optimized by gradient PCR), 1min

Extension- 72°C, 2 min)

Final extension- 72°C, 10 min

Holding- 4°C

35-40 cycles

After completion of PCR, loading dye is added to the sample and agarose gel electrophoresis is performed.

Result

The different samples are compared on the basis of number and size of fragments generated. The RAPD pattern generated are the genetic fingerprint of that organism and are the basis of molecular phylogenetic relationship.

DNA-DNA Hybridization

Principle

DNA-DNA hybridization is a process of annealing of two complementary single stranded DNA sequences to form a double stranded hybrid. In microbiology this technique is used to trace evolutionary relationships between related or non related species. Since DNA is the carrier of genetic information any change in the genome during evolution will be reflected in the base pair sequences. Therefore evolutionary relationship is estimated by comparing the level of similarity or dissimilarity of sequences between species. Therefore more similar the species, more percentage of hybrids would be formed and vice versa.

Materials Required

1. Purified DNA of species.
2. Heat bath
3. Spectrophotometer

Method

1. Genomic DNA of the compairing species has to be isolated using appropriate protocol.
2. The DNA is partially digested to smaller fragments (500-1000 bp)
3. The DNA samples are slowly heated to 90°C to denature the double stranded fragments.

4. The single strand of species A and species B are mixed together and allowed to cool slowly. This allows renaturation of single stranded DNA to form DNA-DNA hybrids.
5. To estimate the amount of hybridization a simple spectrophotometric method is used. The basic principle followed here is the ability of single strands of DNA to absorb more UV light than double stranded DNA.
6. Therefore the DNA hybrids are again heated slowly to release the single strands and simultaneously quantified using UV spectrophotometer.

Result

If Species A and Species B are highly related, then they would form a large number of double stranded hybrids as a result the sample will absorb less amount of UV light. Whereas if species are more dissimilar, less number of hybrids are produced and most of the unrelated sequences would remain single stranded. Therefore this type of sample would absorb more UV light.

When the related samples are heated, they would denature at around the same temperature of 90°C due to extensive complementary base pairing between similar sequences of related species. But the melting temperature would be low if the species are unrelated as the number of hybrids would be low as well as the base pairing would not be strong. Therefore if a thermal denaturation experiment is performed, the related species would slowly absorb UV due to slow denaturation of strong hybrids, whereas the unrelated species would show a high rate of UV absorption due to presence of high number of single strands.

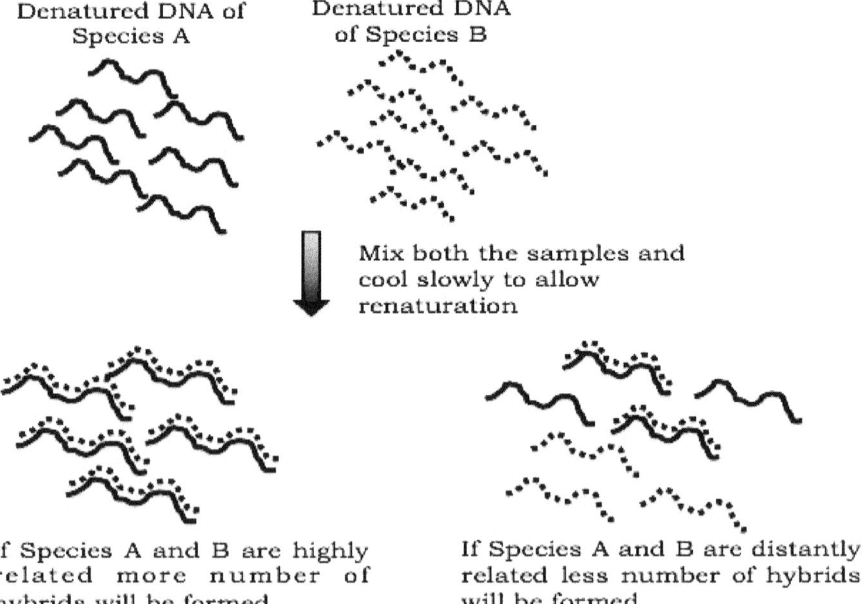

Fig. 11.2: Schematic representation of DNA-DNA hybridization technique.

16S rRNA Sequencing

Principle

RNA is one of the oldest biomolecule which has evolved on this earth. rRNA is present in both prokaryotes as well as eukaryotes and carry several evolutionary information. They comprise of some variable regions which have 5-10 base long unique sequence called as signature sequences whose diversity can be used to classify microbes. Apart from the variable sequences they also comprise of conserved sequences.

In this technique, these variable regions are PCR amplified using primers designed from the conserved regions flanking the variable regions. These amplified fragments of 16s rRNA gene are sequenced and analyzed using several bioinformatics tools. These tools can be used to align nucleotide sequences and find maximum similarity as well as preparation of phylogenetic trees.

Materials Required

1. Purified DNA
2. Reagents for PCR
3. Universal primers
4. PCR machine

Method

1. Isolation of genomic DNA from the microbial species.
2. PCR amplification of the 16s rRNA gene using universal primer set and genomic DNA as template.
3. Purification of the amplified DNA.
4. Sequencing of the amplified DNA fragment.
5. Sequence alignment using NCBI BLAST
6. Preparation of phylogenetic tree.

Flourescence *in situ*- Hybridization (FISH)

Principle

FISH is an advanced technique for genome mapping. This is widely used for localization of specific genes on the target genome. This is achieved with the help of labelled DNA probe that is complementary to the target gene. Both the DNA probe and target genome are denatured and later allowed to hybridize. Following the hybridization step, the fluorescence signals from the probes are visualized under fluorescence microscope. The benefit of this process is that the natural position of the target gene can be identified *in situ* (i.e. within the genome). This molecular biology technique has great application in microbial studies, specifically in identification of microbes from environment samples as well as medical samples. Either it is a microbial infected sample from human or microbial consortia of a biofilm, the microbial composition can be well characterised by using an rRNA probe. It is well known that rRNA has some conserved regions in their gene sequences. Probes can be designed which are complementary to these species specific or genus specific conserved regions of rRNA. Therefore when probes are hybridized to mixed population, they specifically bind to their respective complementary sequences, which could be observed by the fluorescence under high resolution microscope (Amann, 2001; Pernthaler, 2001).

Materials Required

1. Fluorescent labelled DNA probe complementary to targeted gene
2. Microbial sample
3. Fluorescence Microscope.

Method

A generalized flowchart of the method has been described in this section. These steps have to be optimized according to the type of samples and the type of probes to be used.

- The first step involves preparation of fluorescently labelled DNA probes or fluorescent labelling of substrates (if DNA probes are attached to enzymes). This is a highly customized step which is influenced by the type of dyes and substrates to be used. Otherwise customized labelled probes can be purchased, which may be expensive.
- The concentration of the probe as well as quality has to be checked prior to hybridization technique. This can be done by quantifying the DNA probe concentration at 260nm. The quality can be checked by measuring the fluorescence intensity at the respective wavelength of the dye used.
- Next step involves fixation of the microbial samples. The samples could be fixed on glass slides (solid samples) or on polycarbonate filters (aqueous samples).
- In order to enable efficient labelling, the microbial cells has to be permeablized. This could be done by treating the fixed samples with enzymes like lysozyme or proteinase K.
- Post permeabilization, labelled probes are allowed to hybridize.
- Post hybridization, the fixed samples are washed with PBS to discard unbound probes.
- If enzyme labelled probes are used, substrate is added and allowed to incubate.
- Following incubation the samples are observed under fluoresence microscope.

Flourescence Activated Cell sorter (FACS)

Principle

FACS is a biophysical technique used for cell counting and sorting, wherein cell suspended in buffer solution are counted as they pass through a beam of laser. It is a method of sorting cells from heterogeneous population one cell at a time on the basis of cell's ability to scatter light or fluoresce. In microbiology this technique is used for determining shape and size of bacteria, presence of fluorescent pigments as well as community structure.

Flow cytometry systems have a complex instrumentation setup. They comprise of several components like (1) the light source, either a laser or mercury arc lamp, (2) the flow chamber and optical assembly, (3) the electronics that convert the light scatter and fluorescent impulses to digital signals, and (4) computer systems that control the instrument's operation, data collection, and analysis.

Materials Required

1. Appropriate reagents (Refer published research articles for appropriate protocol)
2. FACS instrument

Method

1. The first step in the flow cytometric analysis is to prepare a suspension culture. Most of the microbes appear as colonies or as biofilm or may be attached to substratum. These organisms need to be detached and brought into suspension culture for single cell analysis. Many physical (sonication/ vortexing/shaking) as well as chemical (sodium pyrophosphate) methods can be used for detachment.
2. To determine the cell structure, morphology as well as physiology several mechanisms have been proposed to fix the cells at a particular metabolic state. Fixation is done to either block membrane to prevent leakage of stains, or to block protein synthesis or to block RNA content. Fixing can be done by treatment with several chemicals like formaldehyde, glutraldehyde, ethanol, sodium azide, metal ions or a combination of these chemicals. The method of fixing varies on the basis of cell types and purpose of analysis.
3. Cell Size Analysis: Light scattering occurs when a particle deflects incident laser light. The extent to which this occurs depends on the size and internal complexity. Cell shape and surface topography are critical factors affecting total light scatter. In Flow cytometry, Forward-scattered light (FSC) is proportional to cell-surface area or size. Forward scattered light is detected in front of the incident laser beam trajectory by a photodiode or by a photomultiplier tube (PMT)
4. Internal Complexity Analysis: Cell granularity, protein content, dry weight or any other internal complexity of the cell can be measured by side scattered light. Any change in the refractive index within the cell leads to refraction and reflection of light. SSC measures this refracted and reflected light and it is collected at approximately 90 degrees to the laser beam by a collection lens and then redirected by a beam splitter to the appropriate detector.
5. Cell cycle analysis: Cell cycle analysis can be done using flow cytometry by quantitation of DNA content. The DNA of bacterial cells is stained

by appropriate DNA binding dyes. These dye follow a stoichiometric, i.e. they bind in proportion to the amount of DNA present in the cell. The cells having higher DNA content will take up proportionally more dye and will fluoresce more brightly. For this analysis the cells are first harvested and washed in PBS. They are fixed in cold 70% ethanol for 30 min at 4°C. The fixed samples are washed twice with PBS. RNA content in the cell is removed by addition of ribonuclease. This will ensure only DNA, not RNA, is stained. Finally appropriate DNA binding dye is added and samples are analyzed by flow cytometry.

6. Delection Using Fluorochromes: In flow cytometry optical system the argon ion laser is commonly used as it emits 488-nm light which can excite multiple fluorochromes. Fluorescein isothiocyanate (FITC) is one such fluorochrome whose absorption spectrum is close to 488-nm. Multiple fluorochromes can be used simultaneously if each of their excitation wavelength is near to 488 nm and their emission wavelength is not very close to each other. Any microbe possessing any fluorescent compound or tagged with any fluorochrome can be detected using this method. The amount of fluorescent signal detected is proportional to the number of fluorochrome molecules on the microbe.

High Resolution Melting Curve Analysis for Species Identification

Principle

Melting temperature (T_m) may be defined as the temperature at which half of the double stranded DNA is in single stranded form. The T_m value is sequence specific. It primarily depends on the nucleotide composition of the sequence. High Resolution Melting (HRM) analysis is a relatively new, post-PCR analysis method used to identify variations in nucleic acid sequences like mutations, polymorphisms and epigenetic differences in double-stranded DNA samples. HRM analysis is based on the dissociation behavior of dsDNA due to increasing temperature. Melting of dsDNA depends on its GC content and overall distribution of bases. Melting curve analysis is a technique for analyzing the dissociation-characteristics of double-stranded DNA during heating which leads to increase in the absorbance intensity (hyperchromicity). In HRM a PCR product is generated through amplification and is then subjected to a gradual temperature increase. This is done in the presence of a dye that fluoresces when bound to double-stranded DNA (Tong & Giffard, 2012).

Materials Required

1. PCR master mix with intercalating dye
2. Primers specific to target gene
3. Real Time-PCR

Method

1. The first step is designing of primers for amplification.
2. The PCR master mix comprises of special saturation dyes known as

intercalating dyes that fluoresce only in the presence of double stranded DNA.

3. The region of interest within the DNA sequence is first amplified using the polymerase chain reaction. The region of interest amplified is known as amplicon.
4. As the amplicon concentration in the reaction tube increases the fluorescence exhibited by the double stranded amplified product also increases.
5. The second part of the reaction is HRM analysis. In this process the amplicon is heated around 50°C-95°C. As the temperature increases, gradually the fluorescence declines and as the amplicon completely denatures the fluorescence fades away. The fluorescence data obtained is plotted verses the increasing temperature, generating a Melting Curve.
6. Different genetic sequences melt at different rates. Even a very small change like SNPs in the sample DNA sequence will create differences in the HRM curve.
7. Using this technique genotype of microbial species can be identified. Different species would generate distinguishable melting profiles based on their different Tm values. A single gene like 16s rRNA or multiple genes can be used for bacterial identification using HRM technique.

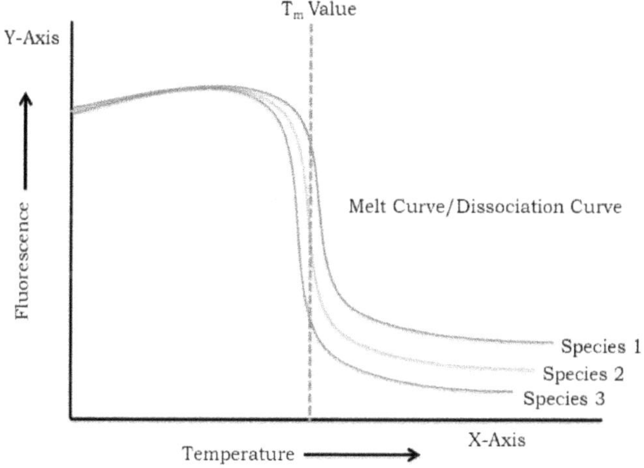

Fig. 11.3: Melt Curve (Tm Curve)

Estimation of GC Content

Principle

The genome of any organism is composed of four nucleotides i.e. A,T,G,C. They have a specific hydrogen bonding where A binds to T through two hydrogen bonds and G binds to C through 3 hydrogen bonds. GC content also known as GC ratio or G+C ratio is the percentage of nitrogen bases in the genome that are either G or C. The GC ratio, the organisms is highly variable. They range from as low as 17%

to as high as 75%. In any organism the GC content remains uniform over the entire genome. Therefore GC content of genomic DNA is used as one of the criterions for the classification and identification of bacterial species (Sueoka, 1962).

Materials Required

1. Microbial genomic DNA sample
2. Standard DNA sample
3. P1 Nuclease enzyme
4. Bovine alkaline phosphatase
5. Appropriate buffers and reagents for HPLC
6. HPLC with C18 reversed-phase column

Method

1. HPLC is the most commonly used method for estimation of GC content.
2. The microbe is grown in a suitable media.
3. Genomic DNA is isolated by appropriate method.
4. DNA is desalted by dialysis.
5. The nucleotides are dephosphorylized with bovine alkaline phosphatase
6. The DNA is degraded by P1 Nuclease as per manufacturer instruction.
7. The resulting deoxyribonucleosides are analyzed by HPLC. Appropriate standard DNA having GC content in the range of 40-60% is generally analyzed along with unknown microbial samples.
8. G+C values are calculated from the ratio of deoxyguanosine and thymidine according to the method of Mesbah et al. (1989).

Fatty Acid Methyl Ester (FAME) Analysis

Principle

FAME is type of fatty acids that are derived from transesterification of fats with alcohol. In transesterification process, a glyceride molecule reacts with alcohol in the presence of a catalyst forming a mixture of fatty acid esters and an alcohol. This test is extensively performed to identify microbial species. Different microbes have different fatty acid composition on their membrane. So, on performing transesterification they produce a typical FAME pattern which can be considered as a fingerprint for that specific organism (Schutter & Dick, 2000).

Materials Required

1. Saponification on reagent: 30% Sodium hydroxide (w/v) dissolved in 1:1 ratio of methanol and deionized water.
2. Methylation reagent: 6.00 N hydrochloric acid dissolved in methanol.
3. Extraction Solvent: Equal volume of hexane and methyl tert-butyl ether (MTBE) mixed by stirring.
4. Base Wash: 1.5% Sodium hydroxide dissolved in deionized water.

5. Saturated NaCl: 40% NaCl dissolved in deionized water.

Reagents used are of HPLC and GC grade, freshly prepared and stored at room temperature.

Method

1. The pure microbial cultures are grown in suitable solid media and single isolated colonies are harvested using an inoculation loop. The colony is placed in a sterile culture tube with screw cap.
2. 1.0 ml of saponification reagent is added to the culture tubes. The tubes are vortexed for 5-10 sec and incubated in boiling water bath at 95°C-100°C for 5 min. The tubes are removed from the water bath and cooled slightly and vortexed for 5-10 sec. Following this the tubes are again incubated in water bath for 25min and then allowed to cool.
3. Next 2.0 ml of methylation reagent is added in each tube and vortexed for 5-10 sec. The tubes are heated at 80°C ± 1°C in a water bath for 10 ± 1 min. This is followed by quick cooling in cold water bath or ice.
4. 1.25 ml of extraction reagent is added to each tube and placed on a rotator or shaker for gentle mixing for 10 min.
5. Following this, the aqueous (lower) phase is discarded.
6. 3.0 ml of base wash reagent is added to the tube placed on rotor or shaker for gentle mixing for 5 min, followed by centrifugation for 3 min at 2000 rpm. After the layers have separated about 2/3 of the organic (upper) phase is transferred to a clean GC sample vial for gas chromatographic (GC) analysis.
7. The FAME profiles obtained are analyzed using latest version of MIDI Sherlock software.

Chapter 12

Metagenomics

Microbes (bacteria, viruses, some fungi, protozoans etc.) are present almost everywhere. Bacteria are present in the water that we drink, the food that we take and the air we breathe. Thes are present outside as well as inside of our body. But very less or almost nothing is known about them because of our inability to culture them. Whatever is known about bacteria is based on the bacterial members that can be grown in laboratory. It has been estimated that only 0.1 to 1% of bacteria present in our environment are culturable i.e. that can be grown in laboratory condition (Torsvik *et.al.,* 1990). Rest 99 to 99.99% of bacteria which are not growing in laboratory conditions (at least in present available methods) is known as unculturable bacteria. They fail to grow in laboratory conditions because their exact growth requirements i.e. nutrients, physiochemical environment and growth support systems are not known.

In view of these all problems a new culture independent technique has been developed for identification and characterization of unculturable bacteria. This is known as Metagenomics (also referred as environmental and community genomics). Thus metagenome is the study of all the genetic material present in a given sample, mostly the environmental samples such as soil, water, sewage material, gut microbiome etc. In this technique, all the DNA present in an environmental sample is isolated. This genome pool is the mixture of DNA of different types of microbes such as bacteria, fungus, viruses and may be some microscopic eukaryotic organisms. To identify the bacterial communities present in the sample, 16S rRNA gene sequencing is performed using universal primers (Woese, 1987). Similarly18S rRNA gene sequencing is performed for identification of eukaryotic microorganism such as yeasts.

Metagenome for bacterial identification

Metagenomics has several applications such as identification of novel genes such as bacteriorhodopsin, genes required for antagonism, mutualism, different survival mechanisms, discovery of potent new antimicrobial agents, lateral gene transfer etc. This chapter discussed the use of metagenome for bacterial identification. It is known that all bacteria contain 16S and rRNA gene sequence which is highly conserved and are used for bacterial identification. The function of 16S and rRNA gene has not changed over a period of time and thus random changes in the sequence make it more accurate measurement of evolution. 16S rRNA is about 1525 bp long and contain 9 hyper variable region designated as V1-V9 region and length ranging from 30-100 bp. 16S rRNA gene contains highly conserved region between these hyper variable regions. Total 16S rRNA sequencing or partial sequences such as V1-V3 or V1-V5 etc can be used for bacterial identification.

Steps followed for metagenome sequencing and analysis: The major steps followed for metagenome sequencing and analysis are following-

Sampling

Sample collected for metagenome analysis are generally environmental or of human/animal origin. The samples may be soil, water, particles present in air, plant rhizosphere, animal's viscera, fecal material, any animal or plant tissue, surface of skin etc. The sample can be anything from where we can isolate the DNA.

Collection of sample must be done aseptically. All the equipments used in sample collection must be sterilized and clean so that there will be no cross contamination of microbes of other origin or chemical that can hamper the DNA isolation process. The sample size must be enough to isolate the substantial amount of DNA.

DNA isolation

Isolation of DNA is very crucial steps. Metagenome is the representation of all the genomic content present in the given sample. For metagenome. analysis the basic requirement is isolation of high quality, high molecular weight community genomic DNA. This community includes culturable as well as uncultured bacteria. The DNA isolation method may vary according to sample type and sample size. The sample represents the heterogeneous mixture of different type of microbes. Their cellular structure such as cell wall, cell membrane will be quite different. Cell wall of some bacteria are easily breakable while some bacteria are very resistant towards cell breakage. Applying harsh isolation method may decrease the DNA quality as the DNA may get denatured, whereas applying mild isolation method may leave some bacteria intact and isolated DNA will not represent the overall bacterial diversity. The mild DNA isolation method may also leads to low DNA yield. Also, in the sample some bacteria might be present in relatively good proportion in comparison to microbes that are present in low density or in trace amounts. DNA isolation protocol should be designed in such a way that the yield should be maximum and the loss of DNA during isolation should be minimum. The isolated DNA should represent the genome of bacterial population present in both large amount or in traces. Presently different commercial kits are available for DNA isolation. Most of them use silica-based column where DNA is attached selectively to a solid phase under high salt concentration at high pH. Also the method of cell lysis varies in these kits depending on the origin and source of sample. Therefore they result in better quality and high yield of DNA.

Sequencing

Earlier metagenome sequencing was mostly done by Sanger Sequencing method. It is still popular sequencing method due to less error and longer sequence read (>700 bp). Now, next generation sequencing (NGS) techniques are used for metagenome sequencing for higher speed and low cost. Two popular NGS techniques are 454/ Roshe and Illumina/Solexa.

454/ Roche Sequencing techniques

This sequencing technique is based on emulsion polymerase chain reaction (ePCR) in which DNA fragments is attached on microscopic beads. These beads are encapsulated by mineral oil in water making an emulsion. The solution contains all the ingredients required for PCR. Each water droplet contains a bead which acts as separate PCR unit. Ideally each droplet contains one DNA fragment and one bead. Each bead is placed in the well of picotitre plate and is parallel pyrosequenced. Pyrosequencing produce light which are detected by charge couple device camera (CCD) and are converted in to actual sequence. This sequencing technique produces the read length of 400-500 bp as an average.

Illumina/Solexa

This is based on sequencing by synthesis technique. This technique immobilizes the DNA fragment on a surface and performs a solid surface polymerization reaction which produces a chunk of identical DNA sequences. During polymerization each dNTPs attached to DNA strand produce a fluorescence that is imaged to identify the base as each base produce a different fluorescence. The read length produced by this technique is around 300 bp as an average.

Some other sequencing techniques are also there which include SOLid and ion torrent or ion proton. SOLiD sequencing technique is least error prone but the read length produced is short, around 50 bp which limits its applicability. Ion torrents do not use the fluorescent dye instead it uses the fact that addition of dNTPs to DNA chain produces H^+ ion.

Sequence analysis

Sequences produced by NGS are short raw reads. These short reads need further assembly to obtain a longer contig which is necessary for taxonomical assignment. There are several software to perform this function such as Patric, Mothur, QIIME etc. First the sequences are aligned parallel in such a way that identical sequences should overlap. This overlap region is merged and a longer contig is formed. Sequences are screened based on length and ambiguity and the sequences shorter in length (usually shorter than 275 bp) are removed. Similarly sequences having ambiguous bases are also removed. Duplicate sequences are removed and only unique sequences are kept for further analysis. Now these unique sequences are matched with 16S rRNA gene databank. These databanks contains the information of almost all known bacteria and are updated time to time to incorporate newly described 16S rRNA gene sequences. Some popular databanks are SILVA, Greengene, Ribosomal Database Project (RDP), Genomic based 16S Ribosomal RNA Database (GRD), 16S RefSeq etc.

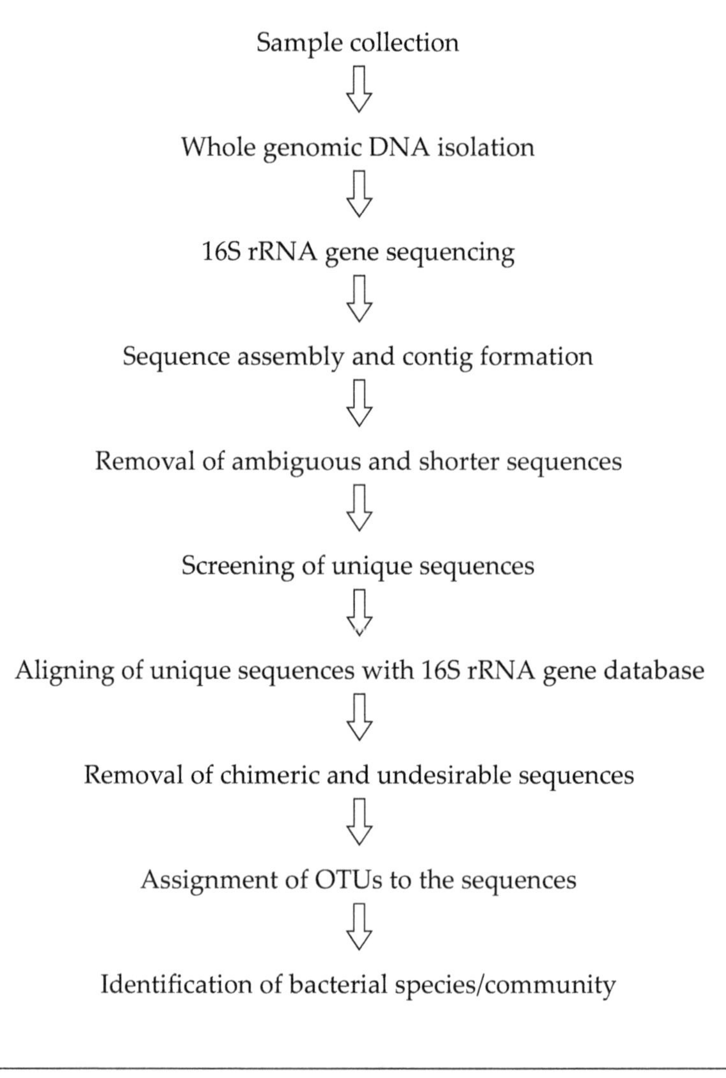

Fig. 12.1: Schematic diagram of major steps in metagenome analysis.

References/Further Reading

Amann, R., Fuchs, B. M., & Behrens, S. (2001). The identification of microorganisms by fluorescence in situ hybridisation. *Current opinion in biotechnology, 12*(3), 231-236.

Bauer, A. W., Kirby, W. M. M., Sherris, J. C., & Turck, M. (1966). Antibiotic susceptibility testing by a standardized single disk method. *American journal of clinical pathology, 45*(4_ts), 493-496.

Clarke,P.H., & Cowan, S.T.(1952). Biochemical methods for bacteriology. *Microbiology, 6*(1-2), 187-197.

Conn, H. J., & Breed, R. S. (1919). The use of the nitrate-reduction test in characterizing bacteria. *Journal of bacteriology, 4*(3), 267.

Corry, J. E., Curtis, G. D., & Baird, R. M. (Eds.). (2011). *Handbook of culture media for food and water microbiology*. Royal Society of Chemistry.

Hajna, A. A. (1945). Triple-sugar iron agar medium for the identification of the intestinal group of bacteria. *Journal of bacteriology, 49*(5), 516.

Harley, J. P., & Prescott, L. M. (2005). *Laboratory exercises in microbiology*. New York: McGraw-Hill.

Herman, B. (1998). Fluorescence microscopy. *Current protocols in cell biology,* (1), 4-2.

Humphreys, J., Beanland, R., & Goodhew, P. J. (2014). *Electron microscopy and analysis*. CRC Press.

Kriss, T. C., & Kriss, V. M. (1998). History of the operating microscope: from magnifying glass to microneurosurgery. *Neurosurgery, 42*(4), 899-907.

Narayanan, S. (1991). Applications of restriction fragment length polymorphism. *Annals of Clinical & Laboratory Science, 21*(4), 291-296.

Olive, D. M., & Bean, P. (1999). Principles and applications of methods for DNA-based typing of microbial organisms. *Journal of clinical microbiology, 37*(6), 1661-1669.

Pawley, J. (Ed.). (2010). *Handbook of biological confocal microscopy*. Springer Science & Business Media.

Pernthaler, J., Glöckner, F. O., Schönhuber, W., & Amann, R. (2001). Fluorescence in situ hybridization (FISH) with rRNA-targeted oligonucleotide probes. *Methods in microbiology, 30*, 207-226.

Schutter, M. E., & Dick, R. P. (2000). Comparison of fatty acid methyl ester (FAME) methods for characterizing microbial communities. *Soil Science Society of America Journal, 64*(5), 1659-1668.

Simmons, J. S. (1926). A culture medium for differentiating organisms of typhoid-colon aerogenes groups and for isolation of certain fungi. *The Journal of Infectious Diseases*, 209-214.

Sueoka, N. (1962). On the genetic basis of variation and heterogeneity of DNA base composition. *Proceedings of the National Academy of Sciences, 48*(4), 582-592.

Thomas, T., Gilbert, J., & Meyer, F. (2012). Metagenomics-a guide from sampling to data analysis. *Microbial informatics and experimentation, 2*(1), 3.

Tong, S. Y., & Giffard, P. M. (2012). Clinical microbiological applications of high-resolution melting analysis. *Journal of clinical microbiology*, JCM-01709.

Torsvik, V., Goksøyr, J., & Daae, F. L. (1990). High diversity in DNA of soil bacteria. *Applied and environmental microbiology, 56*(3), 782-787.

Wilkinson, M. G. (Ed.). (2015). *Flow Cytometry in Microbiology*. Caister Academic Press.

Williams, J. G., Kubelik, A. R., Livak, K. J., Rafalski, J. A., & Tingey, S. V. (1990). DNA polymorphisms amplified by arbitrary primers are useful as genetic markers. *Nucleic acids research, 18*(22), 6531-6535.

Woese CR. 1987 Bacterial evolution. *Microbiological Reviews*. 51(2):221-271.

Zernike, F. (1955). How I discovered phase contrast. *Science, 121*(3141), 345-349.

Index

I

K

L

M

N

O

P

R

S

T

U

V

Z

www.ingramcontent.com/pod-product-compliance
Ingram Content Group UK Ltd.
Pitfield, Milton Keynes, MK11 3LW, UK
UKHW021957270726
14060UKWH00002B/550

9 789390 384587

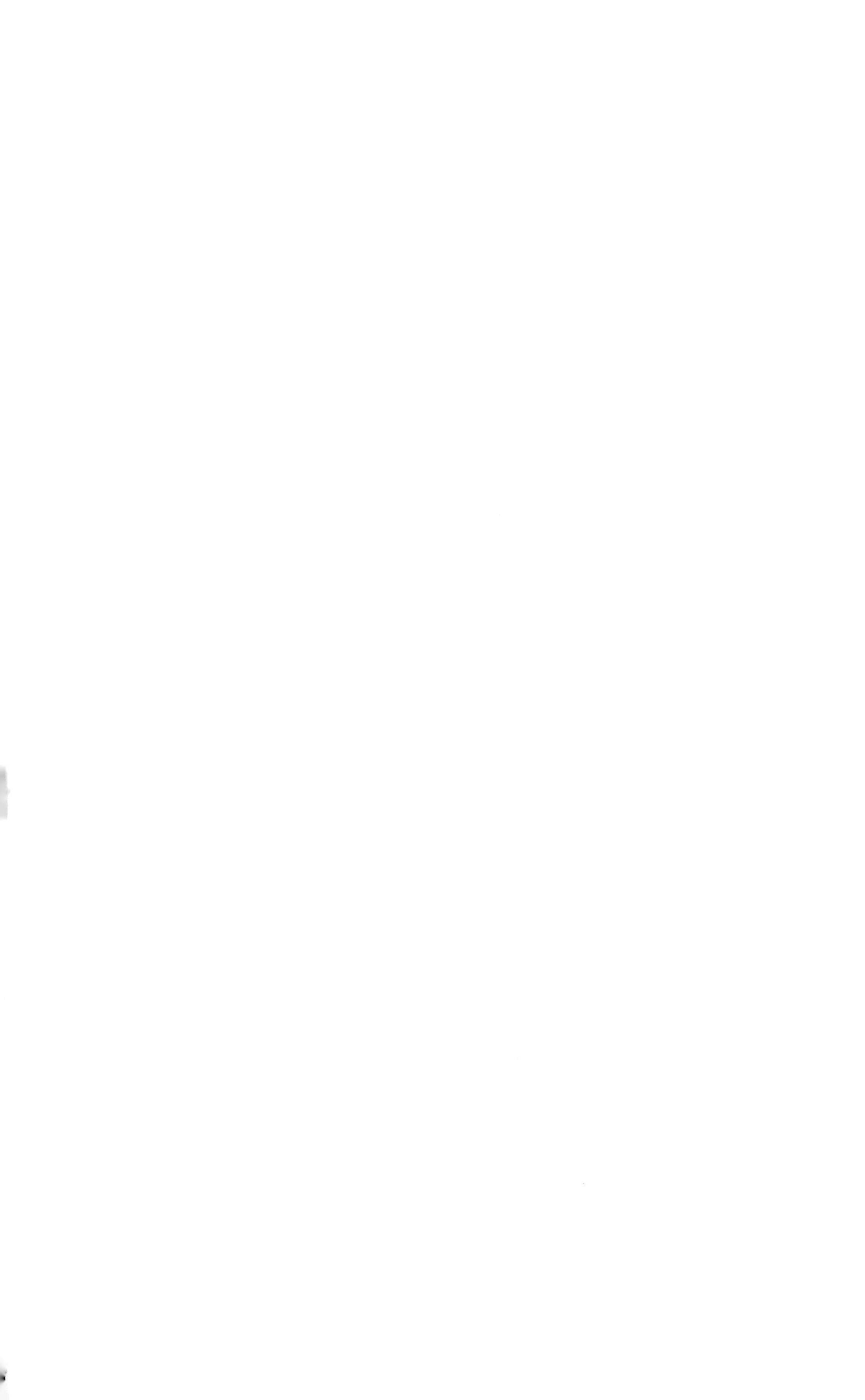